I0031878

AUTISM
— A Handbook of Diagnosis & Treatment of ASD

Sumita Bose

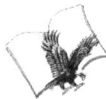

V&S PUBLISHERS

Published by:

V&S PUBLISHERS

F-2/16, Ansari Road, Daryaganj, New Delhi-110002
☎ 011-23240026, 011-23240027 • *Fax:* 011-23240028
Email: info@vspublishers.com • *Website:* www.vspublishers.com

Regional Office : Hyderabad
5-1-707/1, Brij Bhawan (Beside Central Bank of India Lane)
Bank Street, Koti, Hyderabad - 500 095
☎ 040-24737290
E-mail: vspublishershyd@gmail.com

Branch Office : Mumbai
Godown # 34 at The Model Co-Operative Housing, Society Ltd.,
"Sahakar Niwas", Ground Floor, Next to Sobo Central, Mumbai - 400 034
☎ 022-23510736
E-mail vspublishersmum@gmail.com

Follow us on:

All books available at **www.vspublishers.com**

© **Copyright: Author**
ISBN 978-93-813845-4-1
Edition 2015

Printed at : Param Offseters Okhla New Delhi-110020

Dedication

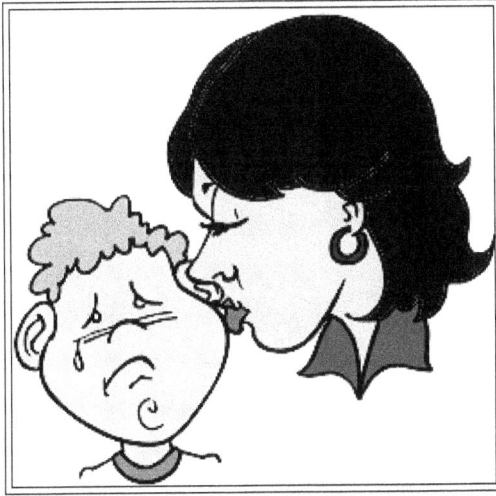

To all children with autism and the people who understand, accept and love them.

"A child is a blessing,
A gift from heaven above,
A precious little angel,
To cherish and to love."

Preface

One pleasant morning in late nineties while working in a school in Delhi I got the news that one of my favourite colleague – Arushi, has delivered a baby boy. Soon me and my other colleagues went to meet the baby. We saw an adorable chubby baby with curly hair, fair complexion and sparkling eyes.

Arushi joined back work after three months of maternity leave. I kept myself update by knowing about the developments of the child. After about another three months, one day Arushi told me that there was something different about Rohit (Arushi's son). He did not respond to his name, did not look at her or her husband when they called him. I asked her "Are you sure Rohit does not have any hearing problem?" To that she told me "No, his hearing seems to be fine since he listens to music and enjoys it too." Then I jokingly told her may be he will become a great musician like Tansen so he concentrates on music and not on spoken words but advised her to talk to Rohit's pediatrician.

Next week she told me that the pediatrician has referred them to the neurologist, psychologist as well as the psychiatrist. Rohit went through a series of tests and was finally diagnosed with autism. That was the first time when I heard the word autism. Worried and surprised I asked her what it meant, what needs to be done etc. She told me that she herself did not know much about it. The only thing she knew was that it was not curable across the world.

In order to help her I went to several book stores to look for a book on autism but could not find any. Most of the booksellers were surprised to hear the word autism. Internet was in its infant stage so there wasn't an easy access to it. I was feeling extremely helpless. The only thing I could do then was to give moral support to Arushi.

At that time I wished if I could travel to Europe or USA and acquire some knowledge on psychology and Autism it would be wonderful. My wish was fulfilled several years later. In 2009, I did a child psychology course from Vermont, USA. It helped me to better understand the children in general but it was not enough to understand the unique children with ASD. So in 2012, I did my studies on autism from the autism society of Maryland. In 2013, I did a autism training course from Illinois University. In 2014, I did a course on "Working with students with special educational needs" and became an Autism Ambassador in Melbourne, Florida. I am currently a member of Autism Society of America.

I wanted to share all my acquired knowledge with the human family of my motherland India. I was thinking of possible ways of sharing my experiences with families back home when miraculously Mr. Sahil Gupta suggested writing a book on Autism. It was a dream come true. The best way to reach people is through the books. At once I agreed and started writing. I am grateful to him for providing valuable suggestions for improvement of the book.

In my book I made an effort to understand the differently abled children. According to the general norm it is believed that they cannot socialize, cannot communicate properly, cannot follow instructions etc. In my experience I feel it is not them but we. We fail to realize their skills and potentials. We fail to understand them properly and become judgmental.

It is rightly said by **Einstein**- *"Everybody is a genius but if you judge a fish by its ability to climb a tree, it will live its whole life believing that it is stupid."*

I have tried my best to share my knowledge and make every child a winner.

I am thankful to the editonal team of V & S Publishers for setting the quality standard for publication and making this book a success.

As there is always a scope for improvement I would request you to spend five minutes of your time in filling the survey form at the end of the book with your suggestions and query and send it to V & S Publishers.

— Sumita Bose

Contents

Introduction

A survey conducted in India by International Clinical Epidemiology Network Trust in partnership with various reputed medical institutions of India found the autism prevalence rate of 1 in 66 children in the age group of 2 – 9 years. The study was conducted on a total of 4000 children selecting from rural area of Palwal, Haryana, urban area of Hyderabad, Andhra Pradesh, hilly area of Kangra, Himachal Pradesh, tribal area of Anugul, Odisha and coastal area of Goa.

Although the prevalence rate is alarmingly high yet very few people know this neuro developmental disorder by its name or signs and symptoms. Diagnosis is often delayed as many doctors treat the children as "slow" or "mentally retarded" or "schizophrenic". Since 90% of the brain develops by age five, early diagnosis followed by immediate intervention is extremely important.

The first and foremost thing of early diagnosis is the mass awareness. It is aptly said by psychologist Nathaneil Branden – *"The first step towards change is awareness. The second step is acceptance."* The parents, grand parents, caregivers, teachers and doctors need to be aware of the developmental milestones as well as the warning signs.

In this book I have provided not only the warning signs and the expected developmental milestones but also other informative text which will answer many common questions which the parents have in their mind after the diagnosis of ASD in their child.

One of the parent's once commented "My entire world came to a standstill when I got to know the difficulties a person could have with autism." No doubt autism is a challenge but it is not a life sentence. It is life with a difference.

This book covers all the areas the parents would like to know about like causes, treatment, education, career and many more things. It is meant not only for the parents whose children are diagnosed with autism but also for the doctors, therapists, special education teachers and those who have their loved ones with ASD.

In this book I have tried to provide the most up to date facts and information. In many chapters I have provided guidance and practical tips from my experience. I hope those will be useful to you.

In this book, I have extensively referred examples from All India Institutes of Medical Sciences (A.I.I.M.S), New Delhi. This is not a media promotional issue, but in my opinion, A.I.I.M.S offers the best diagnostic treatment related to autism in India, and comparable to what is available in the most advanced medical centers in the world.

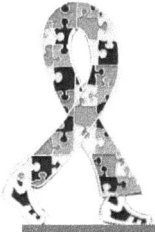

Chapter 1

What is ASD?

Understanding Autism

A group of developmental brain disorders is collectively known as PDDs (Pervasive Developmental Disorders) or ASDs (Autistic Spectrum Disorders). The spectrum of a rainbow consists of a band of seven different colours of varying wavelength. Similarly, the spectrum of ASD represents the wide level of skills, impairment and symptoms. These may range from mild to severe. The characteristics vary across the children and within an individual over a period of time.

Autistic Spectrum Disorder is a broad term used to describe any one of the number of medically similar yet distinct disorders. They are:

   a. Autistic Disorder
   b. Rett's Disorder
   c. Childhood Disintegrative Disorder
   d. Asperger's Disorder
   e. Pervasive Developmental Disorders Not Otherwise Specified

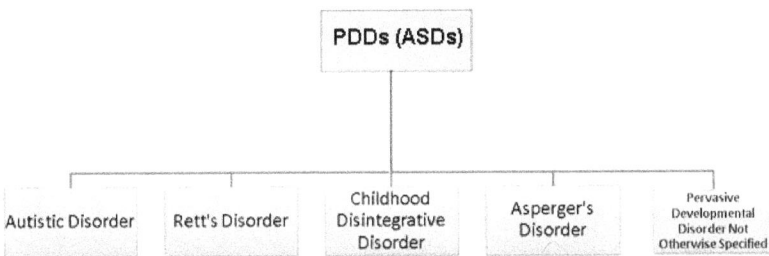

```
                          PDDs (ASDs)
                              |
  ┌───────────┬───────────┬───────────┬───────────┬───────────┐
Autistic   Rett's      Childhood   Asperger's   Pervasive
Disorder   Disorder    Disintegrative  Disorder  Developmental
                       Disorder               Disorder Not
                                              Otherwise Specified
```

Different types of autistic spectrum disorder

Individuals with Autistic Spectrum Disorder exist in their own little world. They have cognitive impairment although about 50% of them have above average IQ. Each individual is distinct from the other but they share some common attributes. These are:

a. Impaired social interaction

b. Impaired communication

c. Restricted and repetitive behaviour

ASD is found all over the world in families of all ethnicity, race and socio economic backgrounds. Males are five times more likely to be diagnosed with ASD as compared to females.

History of Autism

The term "autism" is derived from two Greek words "*autos*" meaning self and "*ismos*" meaning state of being or action. Thus, roughly it means state of being absorbed by one's self or self contained.

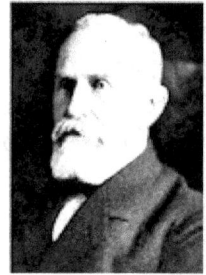

Eugen Bleuler

The term "autism" was first used by a Swiss psychiatrist **Eugen Bleuler** around 1911 to refer to some schizophrenic patients who were self absorbed.

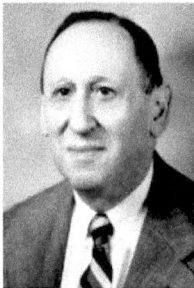

Leo Kanner

Later in 1943 an American psychiatrist **Leo Kanner** found some common traits amongst a group of 11 children. In all of them he found the unusual behaviour and insistence on sameness, social isolation, impairment in language development leading to confusion of personal pronouns and *echolalia* (immediate and involuntary parrot-like repetition of a word or sentence just spoken by another person). He called these children autistic.

In 1944 **Hans Asperger** studied a group of boys and found impairment in social interaction, repetitive behaviour pattern but good cognitive abilities and linguistic skills. This condition is now known as Asperger's syndrome.

In fifties the researchers kept linking autism with schizophrenia. (Normally the onset of schizophrenia occurs during young adulthood. Individuals having schizophrenia often get delusional thoughts, experience hallucinations and have disordered behaviour).

In sixties Austrian psychologist **Bruno Bettelheim** gave the theory that autism resulted due to "*refrigerator mothers*" i.e. cold mothers lacking affection and having an indifferent attitude.

In 1964 an American research psychologist **Bernard Rimland** insisted that autism was neither an emotional illness nor due to refrigerator mothers. He said that it was a biological disorder.

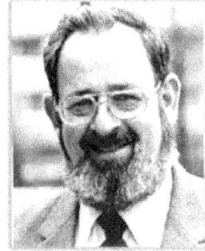

In 1980 autism was categorized as a developmental disorder separate from schizophrenia in the Diagnostic and Statistical Manual of Mental Disorders (DSM – III) the book used to diagnose mental health disorders.

Bernard Rimland

In 1994 Asperger's syndrome was formally added to DSM – IV.

In 2000 a mercury based preservative thimerosal was removed from all children's vaccines (Some researchers said that exposure to mercury in early years could be the cause of autism).

In 2004 the institute of medicine established there was no link between thimerosal and autism as well as MMR(measles, mums, rubella) vaccine and autism.

In 2013 the separate diagnostic labels of Autistic Disorder, Rett's Disorder, Childhood Disintegrative Disorder, Asperger's Disorder and Pervasive Developmental Disorders Not Otherwise Specified were replaced by one umbrella term Autism Spectrum Disorder according to DSM - 5.

Currently a great research is going on all over the world to find the exact cause and cure of autistic spectrum disorders.

Autism in India

Till eighties there were reports that autism did not exist in India. Children with autism were diagnosed as slow learners, misbehaved/disobedient, stupid, moron or mentally retarded.

In 1991, Action for Autism (National centre of autism) was started in New Delhi by three parents, two of whose children received the diagnosis of autism from a psychiatrist trained in America.

In 1999 government of India recognized autism as a disability. An act (Number 44 of 1999) was passed by the parliament to provide for the constitution of a body at a national level for the welfare of persons with autism.

In 2007 India signed the 'UN convention on Rights of Persons with Disabilities' promising to promote, protect and ensure the full and equal enjoyment of all human rights.

In spite of the act and the UN convention there is lack of mass awareness in India till today. Due to the high ignorance level it is often treated as a social stigma. The parents focus more on social identity than on individual identity. Due to the social ridicule the parents hesitate to take their children to public places such as parks, shopping malls etc. They are scared to share their child's diagnosis with their friends, colleagues, relatives or neighbours. Due to the misconception about autism, children are often misunderstood as mentally retarded. It is important that we understand that children with autism are not mentally retarded but they are different.

Regardless of their socioeconomic group, parents of children with autism experience a tremendous pressure from the society.

Although the Indian government and many individuals treat autism as a disability, in my opinion autistic individuals are not disabled but *differently abled*.

In short, autistic individuals are:

A lways

U nique

T otally

I nteresting

S ometimes

M ysterious

Autism awareness

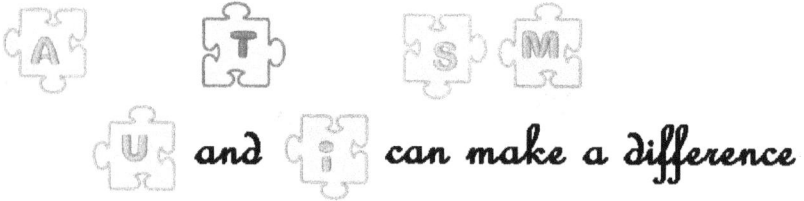

Autism awareness

A lot has to be done to spread the awareness on autism and remove the social stigma from India.

The United Nations General Assembly has designated 2nd April to be the World Autism Awareness Day (WAAD) since 2007 onwards.

Blue is the official colour of autism. Light it up with blue is an initiative to light up historical monuments and important buildings throughout the world with blue light on 2nd April every year in order to spread autism awareness.

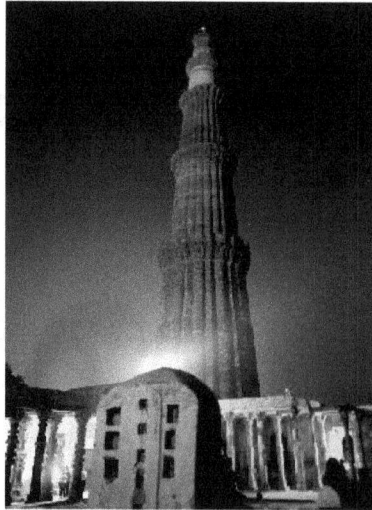

Qutab Minar lighted up with blue light

India actively participates in the awareness campaign by lighting the historical monuments in blue. For example, Agra fort, Qutab Minar, Humayun's Tomb, Safdarjung Tomb etc. are all lighted up with blue on 2nd April.

Each one of us can contribute to the awareness campaign by spreading the awareness in our neighbourhood, workplace, school, college, library etc. If possible, we should arrange for newspaper articles, TV shows, a brief presentation at our local community centre, social media etc. We do not need any particular day to spread the awareness. Every day of the year can be an awareness day. We can spread one fact about autism each day.

The symbol for autism awareness is a ribbon having jigsaw puzzle pieces. The puzzle pieces represent the mystery of autism.

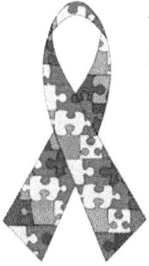

The various shapes represent the diversity of symptoms in ASD.

The brightness of different colours reflects hope. Our motto should be -

Autism awareness ribbon

EVERY CHILD SHOULD BE
A PART OF
THE SOCIETY,
NOT
APART FROM SOCIETY.

In our famous patriotic song "Saare jahan se acha Hindustan hamara" by Muhammad Iqbal there is a line "Mazhab nahi sikhata aapas mei bayr rakhna" which means religious guidelines does not teach us to discriminate among ourselves.

I sincerely hope for that India where love and compassion of the society will not only accept individuals with autism but also give them enough opportunity to flourish.

Autism Statistics

According to the US Centre for Disease Control (CDC), ASD is growing at an alarming rate. The figures are as follows:

2001 1 in 250 children
2004 1 in 166 children
2007 1 in 150 children
2009 1 in 110 children
2012 1 in 88 children
2014 1 in 68 children

In India, a systematic national study on the number of autism patients is missing. There are no definite records (many cases are not diagnosed) of ASD cases. The estimated rate is 1 in 110 children and 1 in 70 boys as per the National Trust of India an autonomous organization of the Ministry of Social Justice and Empowerment.

Some other Facts and Statistics (as per CDC)

- ASD is 5 times more prevalent in boys as compared to girls.
- ASD occurs across all race, religion, ethnicity, geographical location and socioeconomic group.
- About 1% of the world population has autism spectrum disorder. It is the fastest growing serious developmental disability.
- Parents who have one child with ASD have 2 - 18% chance of having the second child also with ASD.
- Among identical twins if one child has ASD then the other is affected about 36 - 95% time. However, in non-identical twins if one child has ASD then the other child may have ASD in only 0 - 31% time.
- Almost half of children with ASD have **average** to **above average** intelligence quotient (IQ).

Myths about ASD

Myth 1. ASD is caused due to bad parenting.

Fact: ASD is not an emotional problem. The definite cause is not known yet but it has been researched that it is a developmental brain disorder.

Myth 2. ASD is a sign that a child is lazy, disobedient, stupid, moron etc.

Fact: ASD is a neurobiological disorder. Hence the affected individuals do not have much control over their behaviour.

Myth 3. Children with ASD cannot feel any emotion.

Fact: Children with ASD have all kinds of emotion as non autistic children. It's just that they have difficulty in expressing their emotions.

Myth 4. Children with ASD have exceptional talents.

Fact: Like non autistic children some autistic children show exceptional talents, some don't.

Myth 5. All children with ASD never learn to talk.

Fact: With early intervention and proper therapies many children can talk clearly.

Myth 6. All children with ASD are alike.

Fact: Every autistic child is unique.

Myth7. The disorders get worse as children grow older.

Fact: ASD is not degenerative. Hence, does not deteriorate with age. With early intervention and proper therapies the symptoms improve over a period of time.

Myth8. All children with ASD are violent.

Fact: Just like non autistic children even autistic children have their own temper tantrums. Since they are not able to communicate properly they get more frustrated.

Myth9. ASD is contagious.

Fact: ASD is not a disease. It is a disorder. Hence it cannot spread by contact.

Myth10. All children with ASD have low IQ.

Fact: Like non autistic children even autistic children have varied IQ level. Some children are even *savants* (individuals with brain disorder but showing exceptional skills in mathematics, art or music).

Autism is treated as a taboo in India. Due to the high ignorance level many parents are unaware of the early warning signs. We need to know the developmental red flags so that there can be an early diagnosis followed by immediate intervention.

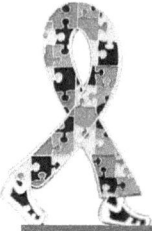

Chapter 2

Symptoms of ASD

The characteristics and symptoms of autism can present themselves in a wide variety of combinations from mild to severe. Long before the children receive the official diagnosis of autism parents suspect that there is something different about their child. Parents should trust their instincts and be aware of the warning signs. At the first instinct the problem should be discussed with the pediatrician who will decide if further tests are required.

The warning signs can start to appear at any age but generally it is seen within the first two years. Having some warning signs does not necessarily mean that a child definitely has autism. Many other diseases have similar symptoms. Let us have a look at the developmental milestones of the infant stage.

Developmental milestones at 2 - 3 months

Expected social and emotional behaviour
1. Smiles back when a parent smiles at him/her.
2. Interested in looking at parent's face.

Expected physical development

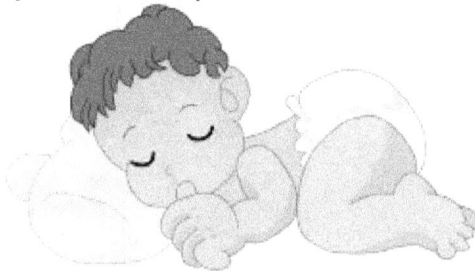

Child bringing hand to mouth
1. Brings hands to mouth.
2. Can hold head up and begin to push up when lying on tummy.

Expected communication

1. Makes pleasure sounds (cooing). Cries differently for different needs.
2. Startles to loud sounds.

Expected cognitive development

1. Begins to act bored if activity does not change.

Warning signs

1. Does not smile at parents and makes little eye contact.
2. Does not bring hand to mouth.
3. Does not react to loud sounds.

Developmental milestones at 4 - 5 months

Expected social and emotional behaviour

1. Cries if they are interrupted during playing.

2. Laughs when tickled.

Expected physical development

1. Follows objects with eyes.
2. Brings feet to mouth.

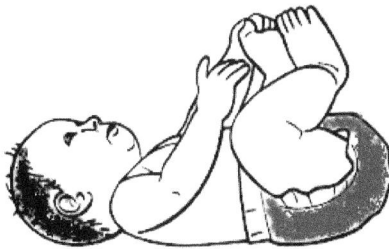

Child rolling from tummy to back

3. May roll over from tummy to back.
4. Sits with support

Expected communication

1. Begins to babble, plays with tongue.
2. Changes sound while verbalizing.

Expected cognitive development

1. Responds to affection with a smile. Likes to be cuddled.

2. Recognizes familiar people. Can differentiate between parents/ siblings and strangers.

Warning signs

1. Does not follows objects with eyes.
2. Makes little or no eye contact.
3. Does not bring feet to mouth.
4. Does not babble.
5. Does not respond to affection. For example, does not smile at familiar people.

Developmental milestones at 6 - 7 months

Expected social and emotional behaviour

1. Likes to play with siblings (brother/sister) and parents.
2. Develops fear of strangers.
3. Begins to express different emotions like happiness, anger etc.

Expected physical development

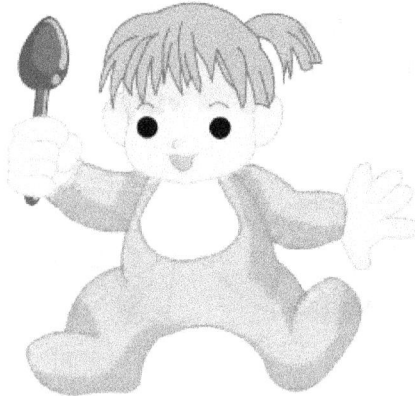

Child holding a spoon in hand

1. Can hold small objects with hand.
2. Can transfer objects from one hand to the other.
3. Teeth begin to develop.
4. Rolls from back to stomach as well as from stomach to back.

Expected communication

1. Respond to their names.

2. Tries to gain attention of others by making various sounds.

Expected cognitive development
1. Begins to imitate actions.
2. Tries to imitate sounds like ma-ma, ba-ba etc.
3. Brings objects to mouth.

Warning signs
1. Fails to respond to own name.
2. Does not like to interact with others. For example, does not try to repeat the sound made by parents.
3. Does not make squealing sounds.
4. Does not try to hold things even when they are within their reach.
5. Seems stiff with tight muscles.

Developmental milestones at 8 - 9 months

Expected social and emotional behaviour
1. Shows fear when scared for some reason.
2. Develops separation anxiety. As a result it has the habit of clinging to parents or familiar people.
3. Shows feelings about likes and dislikes.

Expected physical development
1. Sits without support.

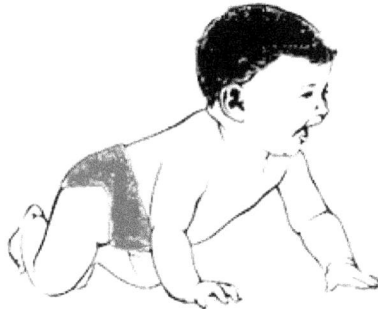

Crawling child

2. Starts crawling.
3. Can throw small objects.

Expected communication
1. Respond to gestures.
2. Tries to imitate speech sounds.
3. Starts to understand the meaning of no.
4. Uses fingers to point at desirable things.

Expected cognitive development
1. Plays interactive games like hide and seek.
2. Can pick up food and put it in the mouth. For example, biscuit.
3. Can wave hand to say bye.

Warning signs
1. Does not respond to parent's facial expression or sounds.
2. Does not respond to back and forth games with siblings or parents.
3. Does not seem to recognize familiar people.
4. Does not move toys from one hand to the other.

Developmental milestones at 12 months
Expected social and emotional behaviour
1. Tries to seek attention by making various sounds and gestures.

Expected physical development
1. Can get to the sitting position from lying position.

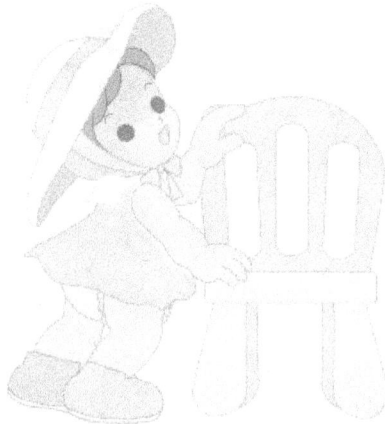

Child standing by holding a chair

2. Tries to walk by holding furniture.

Expected communication
1. Responds to simple spoken language
2. Shakes head for saying no or yes.

Expected cognitive development
1. Can put things inside a wide mouthed container and take them out.
2. Points at objects with index finger.
3. Looks at the right person or object when named.

Warning signs
1. Does not crawl.
2. Cannot stand with support.
3. Does not look at the pointed objects.
4. Does not show interest in searching the objects hidden in front of him/her.
5. Inappropriate laughing.

Developmental milestones at 18 months

Expected social and emotional behaviour
1. Shows affection to known people.
2. Tries to explore new things when familiar people are around.
3. Likes to play with others.

Expected physical development
1. Walks by holding hand. May walk a few steps alone.
2. Drinks from a cup with straw.
3. Tries to eat with a spoon by himself/herself.

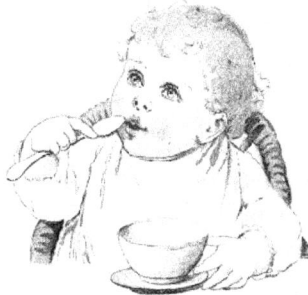

Child eating by himself with a spoon

Expected communication
1. Says single words like papa, mama etc.
2. Learns to say the word 'no' along with shaking head.

Expected cognitive development
1. Learns to point at his/her body parts.
2. Understands the use of simple things like comb, spoon etc.
3. Develops interest in toys.

Warning signs
1. Does not speak single words.
2. Does not walk with support.
3. Does not bother when parents leave.
4. Respond unusually when parents, grandparents or any other person shows affection, anger etc.
5. Uncontrollably repeat words that they hear.
6. Repetitive motions and unusual behaviour.
7. Loses skills learned earlier.

Developmental milestones at 24 months

Expected social and emotional behaviour
1. Likes to play with other children.
2. Begins to show defiant behaviour i.e. like to do what they are told not to do. For example, jumping in water.

Expected physical development
1. Kicks a light ball.
2. Stands on toe.
3. Begins to run.

Expected communication
1. Says short sentences using 2-3 words. For example, papa sit.
2. Understands and follows simple instructions.

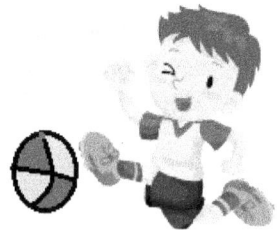

Child kicking a ball

Expected cognitive development
1. Begins to sort colours and shapes.
2. Builds towers with blocks.
3. Names familiar pictures in books. For example, bat, ball etc.

Warning signs

1. Does not say simple words.
2. Does not walk steadily.
3. Does not understand simple instructions.
4. Shows obsession with particular activities.
5. Shows over sensitivity or under sensitivity to smell, sound, touch, light or texture.
6. Laughs or cries inappropriately.
7. Loses skills learned earlier.

Symptoms of autism can vary greatly from one child to another and even within an individual over a period of time. In many cases they achieve the expected developmental milestone till age 15 – 30 months and then start to loose their learned skills. This is termed as **Regressive autism** or **Setback type autism**. For example, children may learn simple words like mama, papa by 12 months then forget the words by the time they are 18 months old. The loss is generally in terms of speech and language, motor abilities, social skills or daily living skills.

According to the research of Interactive Autism Network (IAN), the majority of children tend to lose their skills between 12 – 18 months.

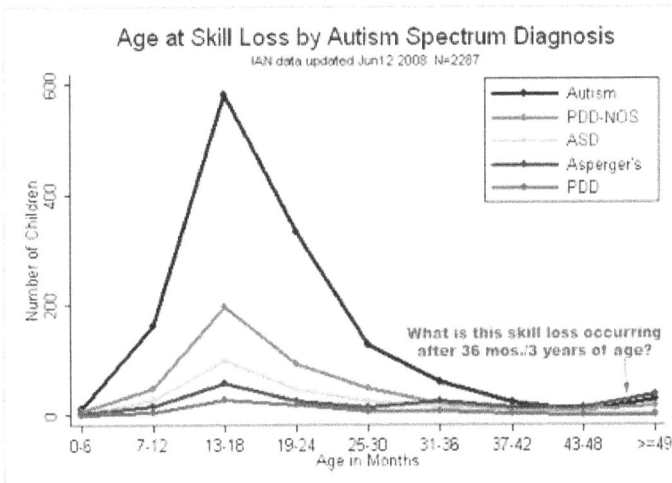

Graph of regression by IAN

According to the researcher Sally Rogers of U.C Davis Mind

Institute there are three ways for the onset of autism –

1. Autism is present from the birth and there is no period of typical development.
2. Regression i.e. the child loses the learned skills after a period of typical development.
3. Developmental plateau i.e. the child reaches developmental milestones for a period of time and then stops acquiring new skills but does not forget the old ones.

Whatever be the reason for the onset of autism we can treat it better if we know the cause.

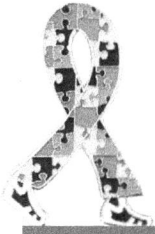

Chapter 3

What Causes ASD?

Around late fifties autism was considered a psychological disorder arising due to some traumatic situation leading to impaired communication and social interaction. Although the psychological cause has been ruled out by the research doctors but the exact cause of autism is still not known. There is no single specific cause of autism. Many things together cause autism. Extensive research is going on all over the world to find the extact cause of autism. As per the current research autism is a *neurodevelopmental* (brain development) *disorder*. The probable causes which leads to the disorder are:

1. Genetic factors
2. Environmental factors

Genetic Factors

Gene is the basic physical unit of heredity which is transferred from a parent to the offspring. It occupies a specific location on a chromosome and determines a particular characteristic in an organism. *Any change in the normal genetic information is called* **mutation**. It can happen without any reason (It can be inherited as well). Mutation can be useful as well harmful.

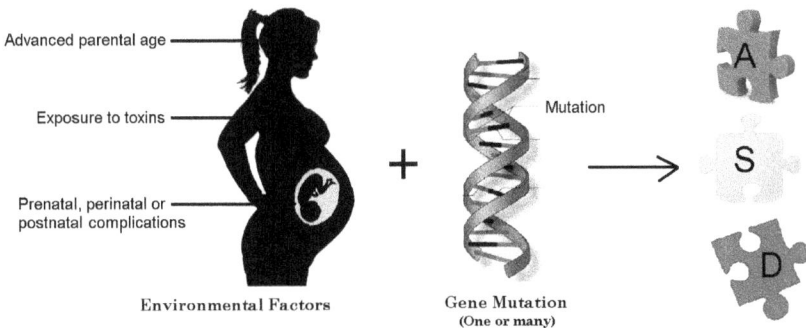

Advanced parental age

Exposure to toxins

Prenatal, perinatal or postnatal complications

Mutation

Environmental Factors

Gene Mutation
(One or many)

A
S
D

Causes of Autistic Spectrum Disorder

It has been observed that many children who have been diagnosed with autism have no family history of any such disease. Such observations and other research work has led to the belief that possibly many gene mutations leads to the risk of ASD.

National Institute of Mental Health (NIMH), USA is one of the largest scientific organization in the world dedicated to the research focused on the understanding and treatment of autism spectrum disorder. According to NIMH if one of the identical twins have ASD the other twin has 90% chance of having it. If one sibling has ASD the next born child has 35% chance of developing the disorder. Although such findings confirm that the genes are responsible for causing autism but the research also shows that many non autistic children also possess some of the suspected genes. This leads to the conclusion that *genes are not the only factor responsible for autism.*

Environmental Factors

In medical field anything outside the body is considered as environment. Certain genes are affected by certain environmental factors. There are several environmental factors which can lead to ASD.

- Obstetric complications
- Inter-pregnancy interval
- Advanced parental age
- Immunization of children
- Exposure to toxins
- Exposure to radiations

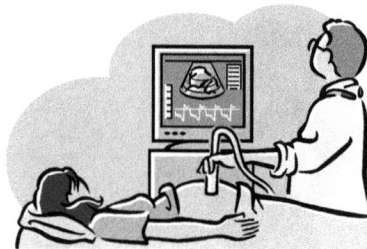

Ultra sound of a pregnant lady

a. **Obstetric Complications** - Viral infections or other health conditions of the mother during pregnancy or during delivery directly affect the development of the child. It can lead to ASD in some cases.

b. **Inter-pregnancy interval** – One of the research studies has found that very short (less than 1 year) or long (more than 5 years) inter-pregnancy interval (gap between two pregnancies) increases the risk of autistic spectrum disorder.

c. **Advanced parental age** – Some researchers have found that the age of either parent during conception is an important factor. The advanced age of the parents increases the risk of getting ASD in children.

d. **Immunization of children-** During the first two years, children are given many immunization vaccines like BCG, MMR etc. This is the same time period when many children develop ASD symptoms. Hence, some researchers connected thimersosal (a mercury based chemical present in many vaccines) with ASD. However, as per the Center for Disease Control and Prevention, USA – "To date, the studies continue to show that vaccines are **not** associated with ASD."

e. **Exposure to toxins-**

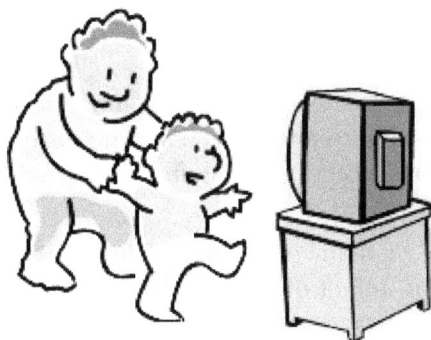

Toddler exposed to PBDE of TV

In our modern world many types of toxins are present in the environment. Some are present naturally while others are released by the factories, industries, vehicles, etc. Many of these toxins are found in our everyday use products. For example, Pthalates present in moisturizers, shampoos, baby products etc. harms the endocrine system. Food preservatives like BHA (Butylated hydroxyanisole) and

BHT (Butylated hydroxytoluene) present in chips and other ready made snacks item causes fetal abnormalities. PBDE (Polybrominated Diphenyl Ether) used as a flame retardant in TV, computer, baby bed etc. has an adverse effect on the brain development. Various insecticides, pesticides, heavy metals like lead, arsenic, mercury etc. enter the human body through the air we breathe, water we drink and food we eat.

f. ***Exposure to radiations*** – The modern gadgets of the present society like cell phones, computer, microwave etc. are constantly emitting radiations.

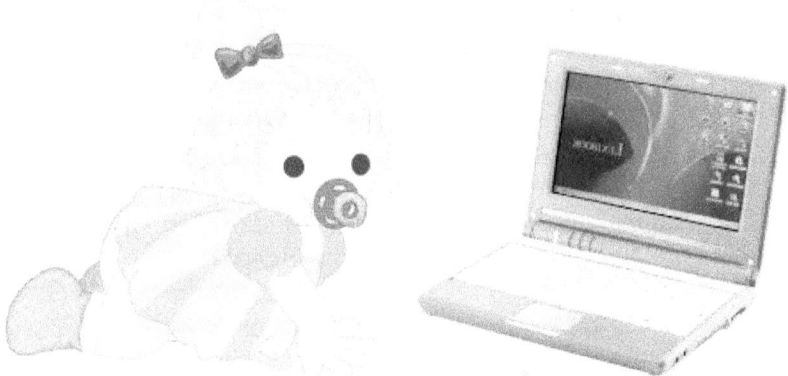

Infant exposed to the laptop radiation

Over exposure to the various toxins and radiations leads to toxic body burden. This in turn affects the immune system, gastrointestinal system and nervous system of the human body which might lead to ASD.

There could be many other unexplained reasons for autism like effect of emotions, effect of thoughts etc. on the child while in the womb. A huge sum of money is being spent all over the world on autism research to find the precise cause and absolute cure. At least at present there is a scientific way of diagnosing children with autism spectrum disorder.

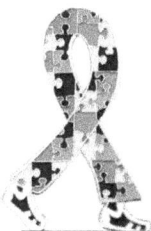

Chapter 4

Diagnosis

Autism cannot be diagnosed on the basis of any medical tests like blood test, urine test, x-ray, scan etc. Parents are often the first people to observe a different kind of behaviour in their children. They should trust their instincts and at the first instance discuss it with a pediatrician. After the basic pediatric developmental screening the pediatrician will refer to the pediatric neurologist and psychiatrist if required.

Diagnosis in India

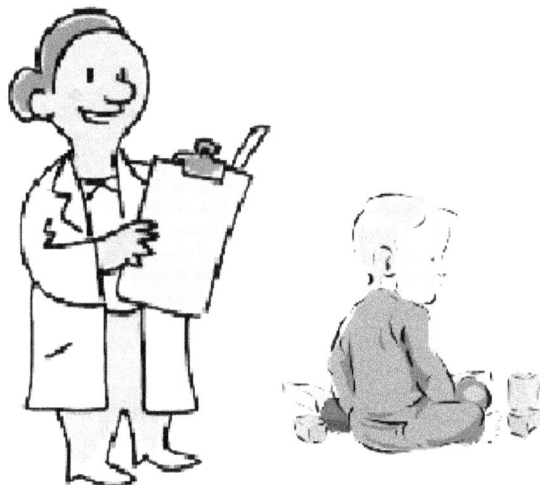

Doctor screening a child for ASD

In India getting an early diagnosis is very difficult. Pediatricians often treat the delay in developments as being "slow". It is troublesome to find a pediatric neurologist. Psychologists and psychiatrists generally certify the affected child as mentally retarted or schizophrenic but being autistic is an entirely different thing.

Autism Diagnosis in A.I.I.M.S (New Delhi)

If you suspect there is something different about your child and you are not satisfied with your child's pediatrician it would be wise to go to All India Institute of Medical Sciences (A.I.I.M.S), New Delhi. They have a separate autism clinic where they do a comprehensive evaluation.

If you do not live in Delhi going to A.I.I.M.S might not be easy. Even if you live in Delhi visiting A.I.I.M.S might be a whole day affair but it is preferable to consult the right pediatrician even though it is cumbersome than to consult a pediatrician lacking the knowledge of autism just for convenience sake. Spending time and money to get the consultation of a pediatrician at A.I.I.M.S will be worth the effort. In case your child has autism early diagnosis will lead to early intervention which will help in bringing out the best in your child.

Patient Registration in A.I.I.M.S:

Address:

All India Institute of Medical Sciences

Ansari Nagar East, New Delhi – 110 029

Tel: 011-2658 8500, 011- 2658 8700, 011- 2658 9900

Web: www.aims.edu

Note: In 2012, A.I.I.M.S has opened branches in Bhopal (Madhya Pradesh), Bhubaneswar (Odisha), Jodhpur (Rajasthan), Patna (Bihar), Raipur (Chattisgarh) and Rishikesh (Uttarakhand). In 2014, A.I.I.M.S has got a sanction for opening branches in Gorakhpur (Uttar Pradesh), Kalyani (West Bengal), Mangalagiri (Andhra Pradesh) and Nagpur (Maharashtra). You can find out whether autism clinic is available at these branches and go to the branch nearest to your residence.

The path to be followed in A.I.I.M.S is:

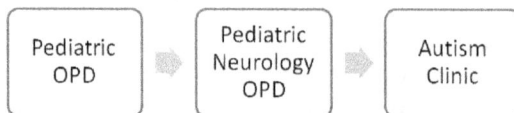

Pediatric OPD	⟹	Pediatric Neurology OPD	⟹	Autism Clinic

The diagnosis of ASD is a two step process:

Step 1. This step involves pediatric developmental screening. Those children who show some problems are referred for additional evaluation.

Step 2. This step involves a detailed evaluation by a team of specialists before the final diagnosis is given. ASD is diagnosed on the basis of the behaviour.

Since there is no pathological or other test for detailed evaluation, the parents play a vital role in observing and describing the behaviour of their child in various situations.

Most evaluation all over the world is done on the basis of the following flowchart given by CDC (Center for Disease Control and Prevention) USA.

Pediatric Developmental Screening Flowchart

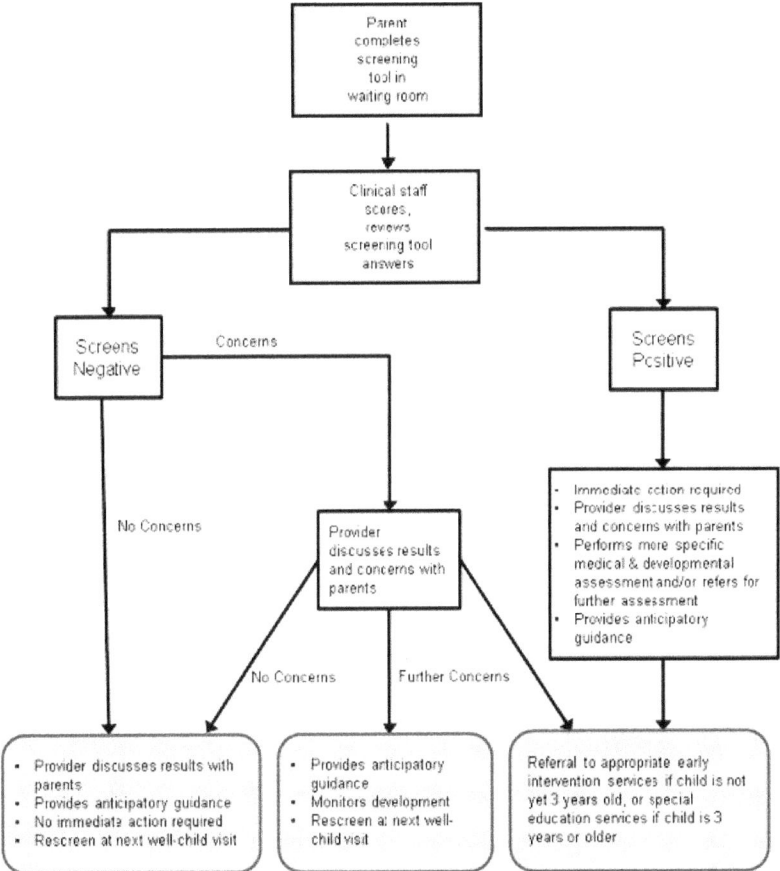

Screening Tools

The screening tools do not diagnose ASD. They do not provide any conclusive evidence of any developmental delay. If the screening test is positive it indicates that the child needs diagnostic tools to identify his/her problem area.

Types of ASD screening instruments (*source National Institute of Mental Health, USA*)

Sometimes the doctor will ask parents questions about the child's symptoms to screen for ASD. Other screening instruments combine information from parents with the doctor's own observations of the child. Examples of screening instruments for toddlers and preschoolers include:

- Checklist of Autism in Toddlers (CHAT)
- Modified Checklist for Autism in Toddlers (M-CHAT)
- Screening Tool for Autism in Two-Year-Olds (STAT)
- Social Communication Questionnaire (SCQ)
- Communication and Symbolic Behavior Scales (CSBS)
- Childhood Autism Rating Scale (CARS)

To screen for mild ASD or Asperger syndrome in older children, the doctor may rely on different screening instruments, such as:

- Autism Spectrum Screening Questionnaire (ASSQ)
- Australian Scale for Asperger's Syndrome (ASAS)
- Childhood Asperger Syndrome Test (CAST).
- Krug Asperger's Disorder Index (KADI)
- Autism Spectrum Quotient(AQ) - Adolescent

Autism A.L.A.R.M Guidelines

In order to simplify the screening process CDC along with American Academy of Pediatrics and American Academy of Neurology has developed certain guidelines. These guidelines are generally followed by Indian pediatricians as well.

Autism is prevalent

- 1 out of 6 children are diagnosed with a developmental disorder.
- The subtle signs of developmental disorder can be easily missed out.

Listen to parents

- ℞ Parents are first to find out that there is something wrong.
- ℞ Parents DO give correct and quality information.

Act early

- ℞ Learn to recognize red flags.
- ℞ Know the minor differences between typical and atypical development.

Refer

- ℞ To a specialist for a definite diagnosis.
- ℞ To a behaviour specialist for early intervention.

Monitor

- ℞ Diagnose other health problems associated with autism.
- ℞ Educate parents and give them an up to date information.

Diagnostic Criteria

The American Psychiatric Association's **Diagnostic and Statistical Manual of Mental Disorders -IV, Text Revision (DSM-IV-TR) 1** provides standardized criteria to help diagnose ASDs. Generally this is used even in India.

Diagnostic Criteria for Autistic Disorder

A. **Six or more items from 1., 2. and 3. with at least two from 1. and one each from 2. and 3**

1. Qualitative impairment in social interaction, as manifested by *at least two* of the following:

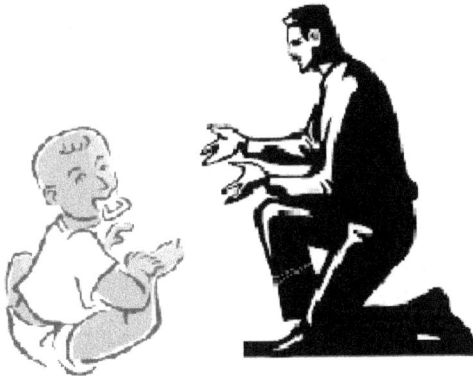

A child avoiding eye contact

a) marked impairment in the use of multiple nonverbal behaviors such as eye-to-eye gaze, facial expression, body
postures and gestures to regulate social interaction
b) failure to develop peer relationships appropriate to developmental level
c) a lack of spontaneous seeking to share enjoyment, interests or achievements with other people (e.g., by a lack of
showing, bringing or pointing out objects of interest)
d) lack of social or emotional reciprocity

2. Qualitative impairments in communication as manifested by
at least one of the following:
a) delay in, scanty or total lack of, the development of spoken language (not accompanied by an attempt to com-
pensate through alternative modes of communication
such as gesture or mime)
b) in individuals with adequate speech, marked impairment
in the ability to initiate or sustain a conversation with others
c) stereotyped and repetitive use of language or idiosyncratic (unique to an individual) language
d) lack of varied, spontaneous make-believe play or social
imitative play appropriate to developmental level

3. Restricted repetitive and stereotyped patterns of behavior,
interests and activities, as manifested by *at least one* of the
following:
a) encompassing preoccupation with one or more stereotyped and restricted patterns of interest that is abnormal
either in intensity or focus
b) apparently inflexible adherence to specific, nonfunctional
routines or rituals
c) stereotyped and repetitive motor manners (e.g., hand or
finger flapping or twisting or complex whole-body movements)
d) persistent preoccupation with parts of objects

B. Delays or abnormal functioning in *at least one* of the following areas, with onset prior to age 3 years:
1. Social interaction,
2. Language as used in social communication,
or

3. Symbolic or imaginative play.
C. The disturbance is not better accounted for by Rett's Disorder or Childhood Disintegrative Disorder.

Diagnostic Criteria for Asperger's Disorder

A. Qualitative impairment in social interaction, as manifested by *at least two* of the following:
1. Marked impairment in the use of multiple nonverbal behaviors such as eye-to eye gaze, facial expression, body postures and gestures to regulate social interaction
2. Failure to develop peer relationships appropriate to developmental level
3. A lack of spontaneous seeking to share enjoyment, interests or achievements with other people (e.g. by a lack of showing, bringing, or pointing out objects of interest to other people)
4. Lack of social or emotional reciprocity
B. Restricted repetitive and stereotyped patterns of behaviour, interests and activities, as manifested by *at least one* of the following:
1. Encompassing preoccupation with one or more stereotyped and restricted patterns of interest that is abnormal in intensity of focus
2. Apparently inflexible adherence to specific, nonfunctional routines or rituals
3. Stereotyped and repetitive motor mannerisms (e.g. hand or finger flapping or twisting or complex whole-body movements)
4. Persistent preoccupation with parts of objects
C. The disturbance causes clinically significant impairment in social, occupational or other important areas of functioning.
D. There is no clinically significant general delay in language (e.g. single words used by age 2 years, communicative phrases used by age 3 years).
E. There is no clinically significant delay in cognitive development or in the development of age-appropriate self-help skills, adaptive behavior (other than in social interaction), and curiosity about the environment in childhood.

F. Criteria are not met for another specific Pervasive Developmental Disorder or Schizophrenia.

Pervasive Developmental Disorder Not Otherwise Specified (Including Atypical Autism)

This category should be used when there is a severe and pervasive impairment in the development of reciprocal social interaction associated with impairment in either verbal or nonverbal communication skills or with the presence of stereotyped behavior, interests and activities but the criteria are not met for a specific Pervasive Developmental Disorder, Schizophrenia, Schizotypal Personality Disorder or Avoidant Personality Disorder. For example, this category includes "atypical autism" - presentations that do not meet the criteria for Autistic Disorder because of late age at onset, atypical symptomatology or sub threshold symptomatology or all of these.

Diagnostic Criteria for Rett's Disorder

A. All of the following:
1. Apparently normal prenatal and perinatal development
2. Apparently normal psychomotor development through the first 5 months after birth
3. Normal head circumference at birth

B. Onset of *all* of the following after the period of normal development:

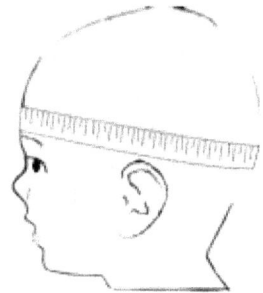

Measuring head circumference

1. Deceleration of head growth between ages 5 and 48 months
2. Loss of previously acquired purposeful hand skills between 5 and 30 months with the subsequent development of stereotyped hand movements (e.g. hand-wringing or hand washing)
3. Loss of social engagement early in the course (although often social interaction develops later)
4. Appearance of poorly coordinated gait or trunk movements
5. Severely impaired expressive and receptive language development with severe psychomotor retardation

Diagnostic Criteria for Childhood Disintegrative Disorder

A. Apparently normal development for at least the first 2 years after birth as manifested by the presence of age-appropriate verbal and nonverbal communication, social relationships, play and adaptive behavior.

B. Clinically significant loss of previously acquired skills (before age 10 years) in *at least two* of the following areas:
   1. Expressive or receptive language
   2. Social skills or adaptive behavior
   3. Bowel or bladder control
   4. Play
   5. Motor skills

C. Abnormalities of functioning in *at least two* of the following areas:

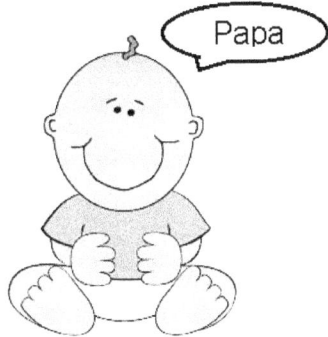

Child showing expressive language

   1. Qualitative impairment in social interaction (e.g. impairment in nonverbal behaviors, failure to develop peer relationships, lack of social or emotional reciprocity)
   2. Qualitative impairments in communication (e.g. delay or lack of spoken language, inability to initiate or sustain a conversation, stereotyped and repetitive use of language, lack of varied make-believe play)
   3. Restricted, repetitive, and stereotyped patterns of behavior, interest and activities, including motor stereotypes and mannerisms

D. The disturbance is not better accounted for by another specific Pervasive Developmental Disorder or by Schizophrenia

DSM-5 Diagnostic Criteria

The fifth edition of the Diagnostic and Statistical Manual of Mental Disorders (DSM-5) released on May 2013 does not classify children according to Rett's Disorder, Childhood Disintegrative Disorder, Asperger's Disorder or Pervasive Developmental Disorders Not Other-wise Specified. It categorizes every child as ASD but with different level of severity.

Autism Spectrum Disorder

Diagnostic Criteria

A. Persistent deficits in social communication and social interaction across multiple contexts, as manifested by the following, currently or by history

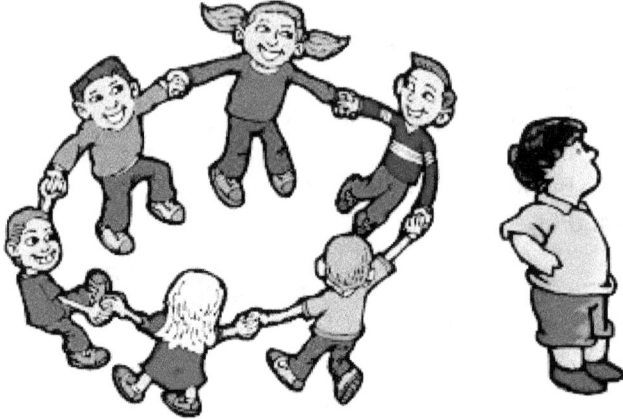

Boy lacking social interaction skill

1. Deficits in social-emotional reciprocity, ranging, for example, from abnormal social approach and failure of normal back-and-forth conversation; to reduced sharing of interests, emotions, or affect; to failure to initiate or respond to social interactions.

2. Deficits in nonverbal communicative behaviors used for social interaction, ranging, for example, from poorly integrated verbal and nonverbal communication; to abnormalities in eye contact and body language or deficits in understanding and use of gestures; to a total lack of facial expressions and nonverbal communication.

3. Deficits in developing, maintaining, and understanding relationships, ranging, for example, from difficulties adjusting behavior to suit various social contexts; to difficulties in sharing imaginative play or in making friends; to absence of interest in peers.

B. Restricted, repetitive patterns of behaviour, interests or activities, as manifested by *at least two* of the following, currently or by history:

1. Stereotyped or repetitive motor movements, use of objects, or speech (e.g. simple motor stereotypies, lining up toys or flipping objects, echolalia, idiosyncratic phrases).
2. Insistence on sameness, inflexible adherence to routines or ritualized patterns or verbal nonverbal behavior (e.g., extreme distress at small changes, difficulties with transitions, rigid thinking patterns, greeting rituals, need to take same route or eat same food every day).
3. Highly restricted, fixated interests that are abnormal in intensity or focus (e.g. strong attachment to or preoccupation with unusual objects, excessively circumscribed or perseverative interest).
4. Hyper- or hypo- reactivity to sensory input or unusual interests in sensory aspects of the environment (e.g., apparent indifference to pain/temperature, adverse response to specific sounds or textures, excessive smelling or touching of objects, visual fascination with lights or movement).

C. Symptoms must be present in the early developmental period (but may not become fully manifested until social demands exceed limited capacities, or may be masked by learned strategies in later life).

D. Symptoms cause clinically significant impairment in social, occupational or other important areas of current functioning.

E. These disturbances are not better explained by intellectual disability (intellectual developmental disorder) or global developmental delay. Intellectual disability and autism spectrum disorder frequently co-occur; to make comorbid diagnoses of autism spectrum disorder and intellectual disability, social communication should be below that expected for general developmental level.

The severity levels (Level 1, Level 2, Level 3) are based on social communication impairments, restricted interests and repetitive patterns of behaviour).

Table - Severity levels for autism spectrum disorder

Severity level	Social communication	Restricted, repetitive behaviors
Level 3 "Requiring very substantial support"	Severe deficits in verbal and nonverbal social communication skills cause severe impairments in functioning, very limited initiation of social interactions, and minimal response to social overtures from others. For example, a person with few words of intelligible speech who rarely initiates interaction and, when he or she does, makes unusual approaches to meet needs only and responds to only very direct social approaches	Inflexibility of behaviour, extreme difficulty coping with change, or other restricted/repetitive behaviours markedly interferes with functioning in all spheres. Great distress/difficulty changing focus or action.
Level 2 "Requiring substantial support"	Marked deficits in verbal and nonverbal social communication skills; social impairments apparent even with supports in place; limited initiation of social interactions; and reduced or abnormal responses to social overtures from others. For example, a person who speaks simple sentences, whose interaction is limited to narrow special interests, and has markedly odd nonverbal communication.	Inflexibility of behaviour, difficulty coping with change, or other restricted/repetitive behaviours appear frequently enough to be obvious to the casual observer and interfere with functioning in a variety of contexts. Distress and/or difficulty changing focus or action.

Autism – A Handbook of Diagnosis & Treatment of ASD

| Level 1 "Requiring support" | Without supports in place, deficits in social communication cause noticeable impairments. Difficulty initiating social interactions, and clear examples of atypical or unsuccessful response to social overtures of others. May appear to have decreased interest in social interactions. For example, a person who is able to speak in full sentences and engages in communication but whose to- and-fro conversation with others fails, and whose attempts to make friends are odd and typically unsuccessful. | Inflexibility of behaviour causes significant interference with functioning in one or more contexts. Difficulty switching between activities. Problems of organization and planning hamper independence. |

Note: Individuals with a well-established DSM-IV diagnosis of autistic disorder, Asperger's disorder or pervasive developmental disorder not otherwise specified should be given the diagnosis of autism spectrum disorder.

It will definitely be a wise idea to consult the doctors in A.I.I.M.S since they use all the latest tools and techniques for the diagnosis of autism spectrum disorder and other behaviour problems like ADD (Attention deficit disorder), ADHD (Attention deficit hyperactive disorder) etc. A.I.I.M.S also organizes parental training from time to time.

The diagnostic tests used by A.I.I.M.S are:

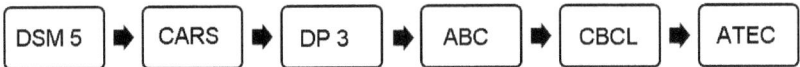

DSM 5 ➡ CARS ➡ DP 3 ➡ ABC ➡ CBCL ➡ ATEC

Test applied	Purpose	Domains assessed	Applied by
DSM 5 (Diagnostic and Statistical Manual of Mental Disorders)	Diagnosis of ASD and severity	• Repetitive behaviour not explained by other illnesses • Social communication and interactions • Symptoms since early development	Observation and Objective assessment by professionals
CARS (Childhood Autism Rating Scale)	• Diagnosis and severity • Periodic assessment on intervention	15 item behaviour rating scale	Observation and Objective assessment by professionals
DP 3 (Development profile 3)	Developmental assessment (Developmental Quotient for 0 to 12 years)	Five scale score: • Communication • Social and Adaptive behaviour • Physical • Emotional • Cognitive	Objective assessment with tools by professionals
ABC (Autism Behaviour Checklist)	• Response to daily life situation • Non adaptive behaviour • Parental perception	57 items for: • Language behaviour • Sensory behaviour • Relating behaviour • Use of body/object	Completed by parents/teachers

Autism – A Handbook of Diagnosis & Treatment of ASD

CBCL (Child behaviour checklist for 4 – 18 years)	Caregiver report of children's competencies and behaviour problems	Eight constructs: • Social withdrawal • Social problems • Thought problems • Attention problems • Aggressive behaviour • Delinquent behaviour • Anxiety • Somatic complaints	Completed by parents/ teachers
ATEC (Autism Treatment Evaluation Checklist)	Measure of the effect of treatment	• Sociability • Communication • Speech and language • Behaviour • Physical health	Parents and professionals

A child gets a comprehensive check up at A.I.I.M.S, New Delhi. Even if the child is diagnosed with autism many parents refuse to accept the diagnosis due to the social fear. No doubt accepting the diagnosis is not easy for the parents but earlier the acceptance greater will be the benefit for the child.

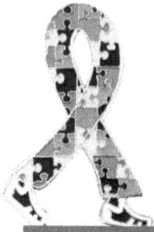

Chapter 5

Accepting the News

If you are reading this book then chances are either you have a loved one in the autistic spectrum or professionally you interact with autistic individuals. In both cases you are a very compassionate person.

In case you are a parent it is not at all easy to accept the news that your child has a life long developmental disorder and realize the fact that his/her life will be totally different than what you had anticipated. Having a child with special needs makes the parents face challenge on a daily basis.

It's normal for the parents and other family members to go through a range of emotions before finally accepting the diagnosis.

Range of emotions after the diagnosis

Within the family each person might have a different emotion after the diagnosis. It's okay to be in grief but the quicker the parents accept the diagnosis the better it will be for the development of the child.

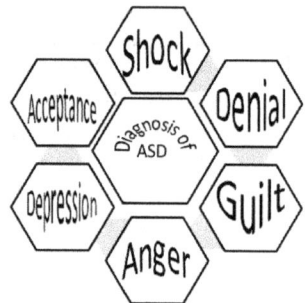

Range of emotions

Shock

Immediately after listening to the diagnosis parents become confused, speechless, dazed or numb. The world seems meaningless and life makes no sense.

Guidance: Give yourself some time to recover. Share your feelings with your spouse.

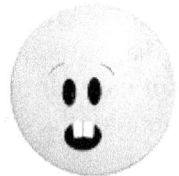

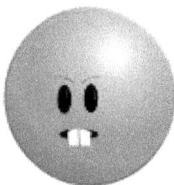

Denial

It is natural to deny the fact that your child is diagnosed with autistic spectrum disorder. You may think of consulting other doctors with the hope of getting a different diagnosis.

Guidance: There is no harm in taking a second opinion. Only when the parent's are convinced about the diagnosis they can make action plan for the treatment and therapy.

Guilt

This emotion is common among the ladies. They feel may be they did something wrong during their pregnancy which could have been prevented. They may even think that due to bad parenting at the infant stage the child developed ASD.

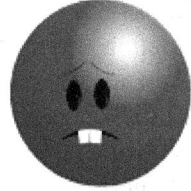

Guidance: ASD is not due to the fault of parents. Come out of your guilt and help your child.

Anger

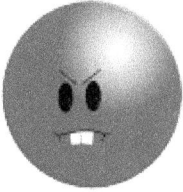

Anger is one of the expected reactions. It arises not only due to the extreme stress but also due to the fact that you cannot control the situation.

Guidance: Sharing helps to calm you. Talk to some friend or relative whom you can trust.

Depression

All parents have high hopes from their children. They have various desires, aspirations, dreams etc. Hence it's natural to feel extremely sad when all these are shattered. It's okay to feel sad but going into long term depression will adversely effect the child.

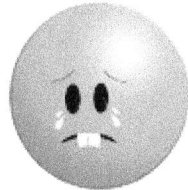

Guidance: It's okay to cry to release your tension. Try to join a support group to get guidance/suggestions from other parents.

Acceptance

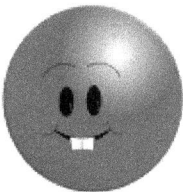

It's not easy to accept the diagnosis of a life long disability. After an emotional turmoil ultimately a time comes when the parents can accept the diagnosis. The earlier the acceptance the quicker will be the action plans for the child.

Guidance: Explore all the resources available in your state (See chapter 26. as well as online resources).

Life has to move on. People can spend hours, days, weeks or even months analyzing a particular situation, thinking what could have or should have happened to them but that won't change the present situation. It would be wiser to find what life has to offer under the given circumstances and start the actions as early as possible to get the maximum benefit. The diagnosis of autism is not the end of the world, it is the beginning of a whole new world. Autism is not a tragedy but the lack of understanding of autism, the lack of our ability to bring out the hidden potential of autistic individuals is a tragedy. There are many famous people in different fields with ASD.

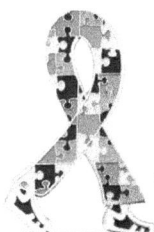

Chapter 6

Well Known People with ASD

Savant syndrome is a condition in which a person with mental developmental disorder such as ASD demonstrates extra ordinary abilities in some specialized field that contrasts with his/her normal ability.

Archeological records reveal that many famous personalities were savant and lying in some part of the autistic spectrum. The diagnostic tools of autistic spectrum developed around middle of the twentieth century. Hence, no specific disorder can be assigned with them but the significant evidence found on the historical records points the personalities towards the autistic spectrum. Some of them are:

Albert Einstein

Albert Einstein the world famous scientist had many signs of Asperger's syndrome (Asperger's syndrome does not cause learning difficulty). As a child he had difficulty with his speech. He repeated sentences obsessively. As an adult he was a confusing lecturer and found it difficult to make small talks. He had problems with social interaction.

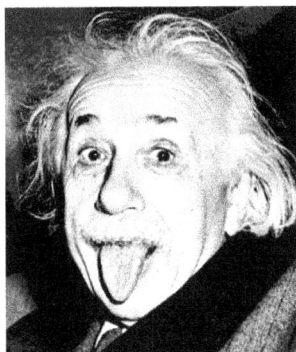

Albert Einstein

Sir Isaac Newton

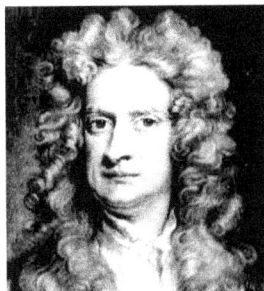

Isaac Newton

Another famous scientist Isaac Newton also possibly had Asperger's syndrome. He spoke very little. He was so focused and engrossed in his work that he often forgot to eat. He did not have many friends since he did not know how to talk to individuals. He followed a strong routine. For example, if no one turned for his lecture at the scheduled time he would still give the lecture to the empty room.

Michelangelo

Michelangelo the famous sixteenth century artist also suffered from high functioning autism. According to Muhammad Arshad, a psychiatrist of Great Britain, "He was a loner, self absorbed and gave his undivided attention to his masterpieces." In his research work Arshad also said, "Michelangelo's single-minded work routine, unusual life-style, limited interests, poor social and communication skills, and various issues of life control appear to be features of high-functioning autism."

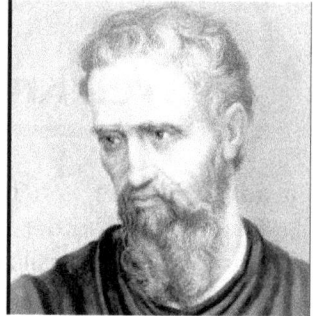

Michelangelo

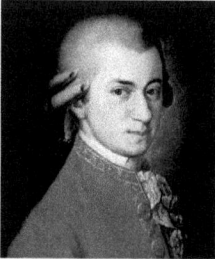

Wolfgang Amadeus Mozart

Wolfgang Amadeus Mozart

Wolfgang Amadeus Mozart was one of the most gifted musician and composer of the eighteenth century. Certain aspects of autism like repetitive body movements, preoccupation with some parts of objects, sensitivity to loud sound and echolalia was observed in Mozart.

Satoshi Tajiri

Satoshi Tajiri is the creator of world famous Pokemon video game series. He has Asperger's syndrome. He grew up in rural Japan playing with bugs. He was so highly obsessed with bugs that his friends called him "Dr.Bug". His restricted interest and high focus on bugs helped him to create Pokemon. His peers at Nintendo describe him as incredibly creative but eccentric and reclusive.

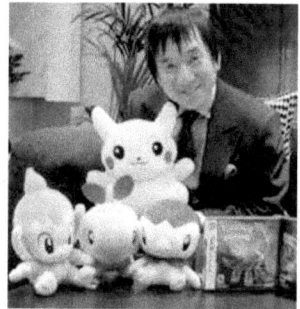

Satoshi Tajiri

Although every autistic child is not a savant but early diagnosis, treatment, unconditional love and support can help every child to lead a better life.

Autism is just the surface, what is inside each child is what is important. Children with ASD can grow beyond their limitations and develop into excellent human beings. It is upto us the parents, therapists, teachers etc. who interact with autistic children to unlock their hidden potential and bring out the best.

It is rightly said by the psychologist Ole Ivar Lovaas – *"If they can't learn the way we teach, we should teach the way they learn."*

We are so distressed with the symptoms that we often overlook the positive traits in autistic children. It is our duty to highlight and enhance the positive qualities of our children.

Fourteen Positive Qualities in Autistic Individuals

1. They are brilliant at concentrating.
2. They are highly focused with 100% attention.
3. They are highly disciplined, hence they prefer a routine.
4. They are meticulous.
5. They are clear hearted, sincere and honest.
6. They give attention to details.
7. Most of them have average or above average IQ level.
8. They are loyal and trustworthy.
9. They have a unique sense of perception.
10. They are not tied to social expectations.
11. They live in the moment.
12. They are good at visual processing work (A visual test was performed by Dr. L Mottron of the University of Montreal's Centre for Excellence in Pervasive Developmental Disorder. The requirement of the test was completion of a visual pattern. It was found that people with autism finished 40% faster than those without the condition.)
13. They are great thinkers.
14. Most of them are good at number skills.

Above all they are **BEAUTIFULLY UNIQUE**. Although there are certain co-occurring health conditions along with autism but good can still happen because the word IMPOSSIBLE itself says I'M POSSIBLE (I am possible).

Chapter 7

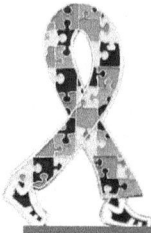

Co-Occurring Conditions

There are many medical conditions and behavioural issues which frequently occur along with ASD. According to the Center for Disease Control and Prevention (CDC), children with autism or other developmental disorders are:

- ⚥ 1.8 times more likely than children without developmental disabilities to have asthma.
- ⚥ 1.6 times more likely to have eczema or skin allergies.
- ⚥ 1.8 times more likely to have food allergies.
- ⚥ 2.2 times more likely to have chronic severe headaches.
- ⚥ 3.5 times more likely to have chronic diarrhea or colitis (inflammation of the colon).

Even though there is no definite data in India but the co-occurring health conditions are pretty much the same.

Some of the conditions that children with ASD may have are:

1. Sensory Problems

Most children with ASD experience the senses in a different manner. They either underreact (hyposensitive) or over react (hypersensitive) to certain smell, sight, sound, taste and textures.

Guidance: As per the requirement of the child use sandalwood powder, sunglass, headphone, stress ball etc.

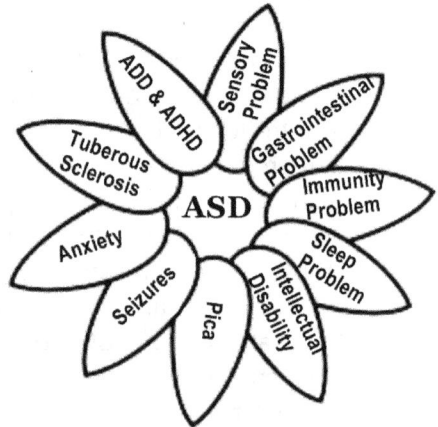

Common medical problems associated with Autistic Spectrum Disorder

2. Gastrointestinal Problems

Many children with ASD frequently get digestion problems which include acidity, stomach ache, diarrhea, constipation, vomiting or bloating.

Guidance: Avoid spicy food. Use fennel seed (saunf) and asafoetida (heeng) while cooking. Both help in digestion by eliminating gas. Chilled milk or vanilla ice cream can be tried for acidity. Give a glass of luke warm water first thing in the morning.

3. Immunity Problems

Some children with ASD have a weak immune system. As a result they develop food allergies and skin allergies.

Guidance: Give protein in every meal. Avoid refined sugar as it weakens the immune system. Increase the good bacteria in the intestine by giving curd. Try honey, it is one of the best immune system builder.

4. Sleep Problems

Many children with ASD have disrupted and insufficient sleep. They have a problem falling asleep and staying asleep.

Guidance: Eliminate stimulating food like chocolate, coffee, coke etc. from the diet and introduce regular physical activity.

5. Intellectual Disability

Some degree of intellectual disability is seen in many children with ASD. They generally tend to have language and cognitive disabilities.

Guidance: Use picture cards and Applied Behaviour Analysis technique (Refer Chapter 11).

6. Pica

Pica is the habit of eating non nutritive or non edible substance for example, ice, chalk, clay, plaster, paper etc. All children have this habit in their initial years but children with ASD tend to continue the habit even after 3-4 years.

Guidance: Pica is an indication of nutritional deficiency. For example, licking chalk or plastered wall indicates calcium deficiency, licking ice indicates iron deficiency. Give

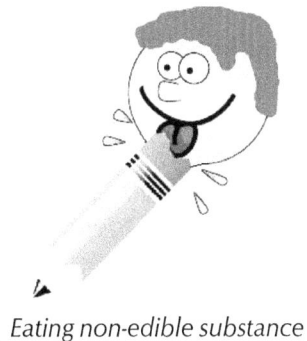

Eating non-edible substance

food rich in calcium like milk, yogurt, cottage cheese (paneer) etc. or food rich in iron like spinach, pomegranate, raw banana etc. as the case may be.

7. Seizures

According to National Institute of Mental Health USA, one in four children with ASD has seizures, often starting in early childhood or during teenage. Seizures caused by abnormal electrical activity in the brain can result in

- ※ A short term loss of consciousness
- ※ Convulsions
- ※ Staring spells

Guidance: The common triggers are flashing bright light, emotional stress, high fever, medicine side effect and sleep deprivation. Avoid them as far as possible. Talk to the pediatrician to see if your child needs anticonvulsant (Refer Chapter 10)

Caution

a. Do not try to put something into the mouth during seizure.
b. Do not touch or hold the tongue during seizure.
c. Do not try to stop the movements of the seizure.
d. Do not give any oral medicine during the attack.
e. Loosen clothes specially around the neck.
f. After the seizure make the person lie on his/her side.

8. Anxiety Disorder

This is a serious problem with many children. It can range from mild to severe. This results in social phobia, extreme fear, mood fluctuation etc.

Guidance: Try various relaxation techniques like breathing exercise, aroma therapy, music therapy, mudra therapy etc. (Refer Chapter 19). Sometimes but not always medication like SSRI needs to be given with doctor's approval (Refer Chapter 10).

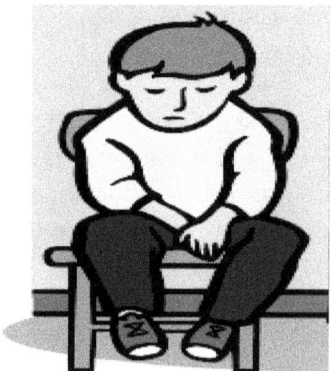

An anxious boy

9. Tuberous Sclerosis

This is not very common. According to National Institute of Mental

Health only 1% to 4% children with ASD get Tuberous Sclerosis. This is a rare genetic disorder that causes growth of non cancerous tumours.

Guidance: Discuss with your child's pediatrician if sirolimus (Rapamune) or everolimus (Zortress) can be used to reduce the symptoms.

10. ADD and ADHD

Most children with ASD have problem with focusing. Hence ADD (Attention deficit disorder) and ADHD (Attention deficit hyperactive disorder) are common in them. Sometimes it leads to their aggressive behaviour.

Guidance: Avoid soft drinks, toffees, fast food like burger, pizza etc. Try breathing exercise, mudra therapy, aroma therapy etc.(Refer Chapter 19). Ask the pediatrician if methylphenidate will benefit your child.

Due to several medical conditions, children with ASD may also suffer from general pain in any part of the body. It is difficult for the child to express the pain due to language and communication problem. It is difficult for the parents to understand their pain as well since the children do not have any change in their facial expression. Even if they can speak there is no change in their tone. So how do we understand them? Although many doctors say that autistic children do not feel pain but I don't agree to this. They may experience it differently. Some might have high tolerance to pain. Certain behaviour changes indicate pain in children with ASD.

Behaviours that suggest pain

1. Change in posture. For example, leaning onto something solid like table or lying on the floor to put pressure on the abdomen for stomach pain.

2. Unusual crying, moaning (making long sounds) or whipering (a series of low feeble sound) which may not be accompanied by any change in facial expression.

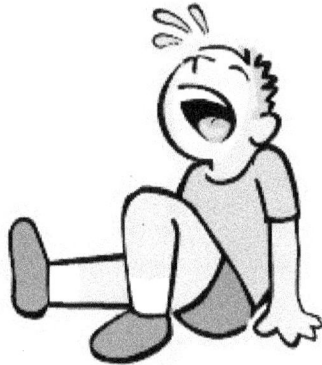

Crying child

3. Self injurious behaviour like hitting head on the wall. This might occur during their headache.
4. Changes in eating. For example, refusing favourite food item.
5. Changes in sleep – may sleep longer or less than usual.
6. Feeling restless. For example, rocking back and forth.
7. Grasping something tightly.
8. Clenched fist.
9. Rubbing some particular part of the body.
10. Does not get distracted with anything.

To make the child pain free and remain pain free we need the guidance from a team of professionals.

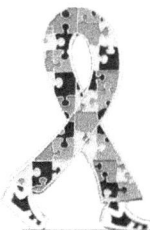

Chapter 8

Professional Team

The time period between the diagnosis of ASD and acceptance of the news varies from person to person. After the acceptance every parent wants their relatives and friends to be supportive but in reality this may not happen. The near and dear ones might be reluctant to support you, they may try to avoid the situation and stay aloof. This should not further hurt the parents. They should understand the difference between their want and need. They need support and guidance from a team of professionals.

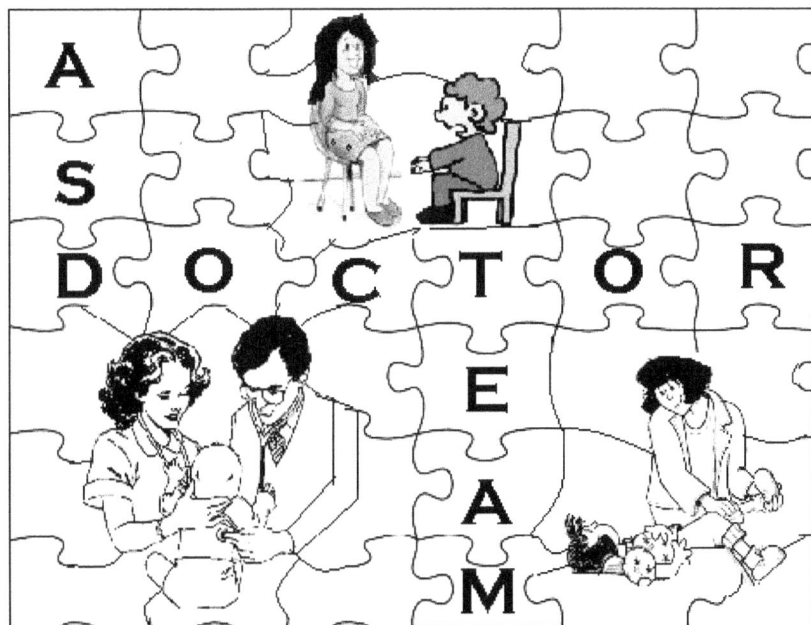

Team of professionals

The helpful teams of professionals are

1. Pediatrician (Child specialist)

He/She does the first level of developmental screening and refers the child to the specialists if required.

2. Neurologist (Doctors dealing with the nervous system)

Since autism is a neurological developmental disorder children having delayed developmental milestones are often referred to the neurologists. This specialist can treat the seizures associated with ASD and diagnose if there is any other nervous system related problem.

3. Psychologist (Mind specialist)

He/she can help the child with social skills and work on his behaviour and interaction.

4. Psychiatrist (Doctors dealing with the mental or emotional health)

The main difference between a psychologist and a psychiatrist is that the psychiatrist has the authority to prescribe medicines. Hence they can prescribe medicines for children having ADD, ADHD, anxiety and sleep problems.

5. Occupational therapist (Specialists helping with daily activities through therapy)

This specialist checks the body coordination and the response to various senses of the child and helps in dealing with the sensory problems.

6. Physical therapist (Specialists helping with the mobility)

Through various exercises, massage, moist heat etc. they improve the muscle strength and reduce pain thereby improving movement.

7. Speech therapist (Specialists helping with talking)

Using audio visual aids they help to improve the understanding and communication of the children.

8. Nutritionist (Food expert)

They help with an individual diet plan eliminating the allergy causing food. They plan the diet based on the various health problems and the calorie requirement of the child.

9. Gastroenterologist (Specialist of the digestive tract)

If the child suffers from regular acidity, constipation or diarrhea gastroenterologist can prescribe some medicine to relieve the symptoms.

At times consulting too many specialists, telling relatives and friend also become problematic since each person suggests something from his/her point of view. This can often become confusing for the parents as "Too many cooks spoil the broth." My advice to the parents would be to trust their instinct, discuss among themselves (husband and wife) and do the needful. Moreover once the child is diagnosed with autism parents cannot just play the role of parents. They have to become education specialist, nutritionist as well as physical therapist. Once they try to understand their child and start thinking from his/her perspective decisions will become much easier.

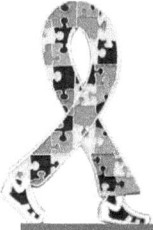

Chapter 9

Know Your Child

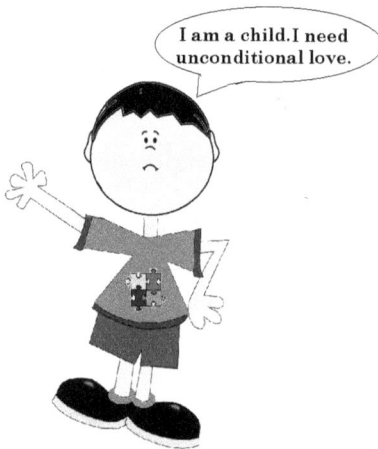

I am a child. I need unconditional love.

Feelings of a child with autism

It is a common belief that children with autism do not have any emotions. On the contrary they are very sensitive and affectionate. They have the same emotions and hopes as you and me. They are often very lonely and want to have friends. The only problem they have is, with subtle emotions. For example, understanding the sarcasm from the tone or understanding the facial expression is very difficult for them. Social cues are just clues for them.

They express their love in their own way. May be we do not see them expressing love according to the way we are used to seeing due to their communication problem and lack of social skills. Mrs. Patel mother of a two year old boy told me – "My son displays his affection by pinching my elbow." The sensory world of autistic children is often very overwhelming. A light hug or a soft kiss from you might be a sensory overload for some children while others may enjoy a tight hug. If it is an overload they will try to avoid you and you might feel that your child does not love you. Be patient and identify your child's sensory preferences then you can use that to exchange emotional attachment. It has to be at their pace, their control and their comfort level.

Let us try to look through the eyes of a child. Every child affected with autism wishes that their loved ones knew the following:

1. I am a child

Autism is just a part of me not the whole. I do have many things beyond autism. You need to understand me. Every person is not a good cook, does not earn high salary or have a fair complexion. People don't hate them for that. It is just a part of them. Moreover my autism is neither your fault nor mine. So let's face it together.

2. Please try to differentiate between won't and can't

Many times you must be thinking that I am stubborn, disobedient or not listening to your instructions. Actually I do listen but cannot understand. So I am not able to follow your instructions. There are certain things which I want to do but am not able to do. Please cooperate with me.

3. I have limited vocabulary

Please be patient with me. I cannot express my feelings properly since I have limited vocabulary. For example, when I am hungry I am not able to tell you and since you don't understand I get irritated. It's very hard for me to express my feelings. Please try to understand my body language as well.

4. Please help me to interact with the society

Sometimes I do like to be left alone but at times I also feel like playing with others. Please teach me how to interact with others since I don't understand the vocabulary, facial expression or body language of others. I take time to understand. I can understand simple things better.

5. Kindly use pictures for me

I can understand things better when you use pictures rather than when you tell me verbally. Also please show me the pictures again and again from time to time to help me understand. I cannot remember everything or for a long period of time.

6. My sensory perceptions are different

My sense of sight, smell, taste, touch and hearing are different. Hence the normal light might be too bright or too dull for me or normal sound might be too loud or too soft for me. Please try to adjust with my senses.

7. I interpret words literally

I do not understand any idiom or difficult word. For example, if someone says crying over spilt milk I will not know that he is complaining about a loss from the past. I will think that he is actually crying since he spilt his milk. I also get confused when I hear similar sounding words for example, red and read or lose and loose.

8. Please try to identify the trigger factors of my emotional distress

I am unable to tell you what causes my distress. Please try to find out the triggers. It could be my anxiety, my physical discomfort, uncomfortable environment, my inability to express what I want to tell you or anything else. It is a horrible feeling for me too. I tend to become aggressive generally when I am not able to take the pressure any more.

9. Please look at my strengths and not weaknesses

Although I cannot do many things as per your desire still there are lots of things which I can do. Please encourage me with those so that I can improve myself. If I constantly hear criticism I will forget even little things which I can do.

Daniel Stefanski, a 14 year old autistic boy has written in his book "How to talk to an autistic kid" – "Laugh with me and not at me. I can tell the difference, even if it seems I cannot."

10. I need unconditional love

I need limitless and unconditional love. With your love, support, guidance and encouragement I may be more successful in life than you are thinking at present.

Parents are a child's first and the most important teacher. There is immense power in love and faith, with your unconditional love and doctor's medicine for treating the symptoms wonders can happen. It is commonly said that-

> "Faith
> makes all things possible,
> Love
> makes all things easy,
> Hope
> makes all things work."

So do not give up under any situation. Your child will definitely improve.

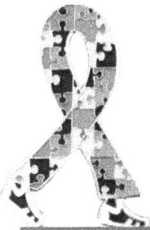

Chapter 10

Treatment

An intensive research work is going on around the world to find a definite cure for autism. At present the treatment of autism is a multidisciplinary approach. There are various treatments to reduce the symptoms and make the child highly functional. Every individual suffering from ASD is unique hence the treatment option for every individual is also different.

The different treatment categories are

a. Behaviour and Communication Approach
b. Dietary Approach
c. Medication
d. Complementary and Alternative Medicine

The treatment categories can be further sub grouped as biomedical and non medical treatment. Biomedical includes allopathy, homeopathy or ayurvedic medicines while non medical includes behaviour therapy, nutritional therapy, mudra therapy, aroma therapy, music therapy etc. In this chapter I will discuss about some of the allopathy medicines commonly used for ASD individuals.

Medicines for General Health Boost

a. Multivitamins

Vitamins are a group of organic compounds that are essential for the growth and development of the body. Many times since the children are not able to eat a balanced diet they are prescribed multivitamins. Sometimes the pediatricians prescribe only individual vitamins.

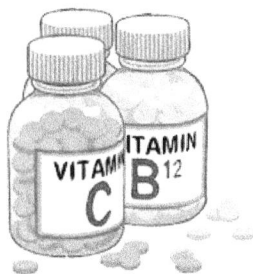

Vitamin B and C

b. Calcium, Magnesium and Zinc

The three essential nutrients for maintaining good health is Calcium, Magnesium and Zinc. Calcium is required by the body for healthy bones, Magnesium helps in the absorption of Calcium and improves the functioning of muscles. Zinc supports the body's immune system.

Medicines for Neurological Symptoms

a. SSRIs

Selective serotonin reuptake inhibitors (SSRI) are a group of chemical compounds used as antidepressants in the treat-ment of personality disorder, anxiety, depression etc. The commonly used SSRIs are Fluoxetine, Fluvoxamine, Sertraline and Clomipramine available under various trade names.

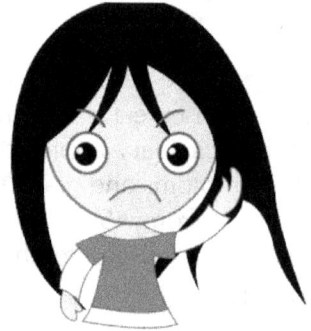
Depressed teenager

b. Anticonvulsant

The drugs that control seizure are known as anticonvulsant. They are commonly called antiepileptic or antiseizure drugs. Lamotrigine, Carbamazepine and Topiramate are the common anticonvulsants.

c. Antipsychotic

Antipsychotics are a group of psychiatric medicines which are used to manage hallucinations, delusions etc. particularly in bipolar disorder and schizophrenia. They are commonly called neuroleptic or tranquilizer. The common antipsychotic used for ASD individuals are Aripripazole and Risperidone. These medicines are useful in the treatment of aggression, hyperactivity, self injury, stimming and other behaviour problems. They also overcome sleep problems which is common in children with ASD.

d. Stimulants

Stimulants are psychoactive drugs which improve the mental alertness, wakefulness, concentration etc. The commonly used stimulant is Methylphenidate which is very effective in treating children with ADHD and ADD. This drug is also effective in children with ASD having similar symptoms.

Medicines for Gastroenterological Symptoms

Periodic bouts of diarrhea or constipation is common in all children, however if it becomes prolonged then the doctor should be consulted.

a. Diarrhea

Mild diarrhea can be controlled by giving boiled and mashed raw banana but for chronic diarrhea the doctor has to determine the cause. If it is due to some infection, antibiotic is prescribed. If it is due to the side effect of some medicine that medicine is changed or the dose is reduced. It could be even due to some food allergy (The child might be allergic to some food which he/she loves to eat).

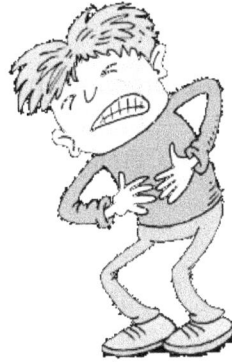

Teenager with stomach ache

b. Constipation

Mild constipation can be treated by giving high fibre fruits and vegetables like ripe banana, papaya, cabbage, potato etc. However for chronic constipation laxatives like Dulcolax or Psyllium husk (Isabgol) are generally given.

c. GERD (Gastroesophageal reflux disorder)

The muscle that acts as a valve between the esophagus and stomach is known as lower esophageal sphincter (LES). The function of LES is to open in order to allow the food to pass into the stomach and then close. GERD is a chronic digestive disorder in which the LES becomes weak and open and closes inappropriately. As a result there is a reflux (flow back) of stomach contents including the stomach acid back into the esophagus. This irritates the lining of the esophagus and causes burning sensation in the chest, throat etc. Medically this is treated with antacids and proton pump inhibitors (medicines that reduce the production of stomach acid) like Omeprazole, Esomeprazole etc.

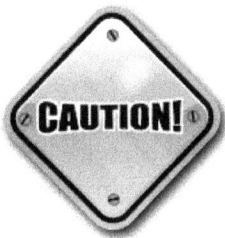

Do not give any medicine to children without consulting a doctor.

All parents need to be careful while giving medicine to children but as psychopharmacologic and neuropsychopharmacologic medicines play an important role in improving the health of autistic children, parents need to be extra vigilant. (Psychopharmacology is the scientific study of the effects which medicines have on thinking, behaviour, mood and sensation. Neuropsychopharmacology is the scientific study of the effects of medicines on the functioning of cells in the nervous system).

Some precautions while giving medicines

1. Always give the exact dose as prescribed by the doctor. Certain medicines work well with food while others need to be given in an empty stomach. Find out the appropriate time of giving the medicine from the doctor.
2. For a liquid medicine measure it carefully. Don't give it by approximation.
3. If specialists are consulted tell them about the medicines given by the pediatrician. In case the child is taking any homeopathy or ayurvedic medicine inform that to the allopathy doctor. **Many medicines interact with each other and have a drastic side effect**. Be careful of that.
4. Store the medicines properly in their respective labelled containers. Some liquid medicines require refrigeration after opening. Ask the pharmacist about it.
5. Do not increase, decrease, start or stop the medicine without consulting the doctor.
6. If you notice some side effect after giving the first dose inform the doctor immediately. Ask him/her if you still need to continue that.
7. Keep all the medicines out of the reach of the child.
   Most children have problem taking the medicine.
   Some of the following suggestions might make your task easier.

Ideas to help your child take medicines

1. Mix the medicine with milk, juice or soup (The tablets can be crushed and mixed. Ask your doctor if the medicine is heat sensitive).
2. You can sprinkle powdered sugar over the crushed medicine and put the mixture over a biscuit.
3. You may try giving medicines followed by a highly motivating reinforcer. For example, the child can be reinforced with a TV programme or a computer game if he/she takes medicine without any trouble.

4. Ask the doctor if flavoured liquid medicines will be a better option for your child.

While giving proper medicine is important, it is equally important to maintain a medical file. In fact, it will be convenient to maintain two files – one with medical records and the other with medical bills and insurance papers.

Some of the important things to be kept in a medical file are

1. Immunization records
2. Pediatrician's prescriptions
3. Specialist's prescriptions
4. Laboratory test reports like blood test, urine test, x-ray, MRI etc.
5. Food allergy (if any)
6. Name of the medicine which did not suit – Mention the side effects
7. Sensory problems
8. Frequency of meltdown
9. Blood group of the child
10. Mode of communication of the child – verbal, semi verbal or non verbal. In case of non verbal what is the preferred mode of communication of the child – through picture cards, sign language or gestures.

Maintaining a medicine chart will be very helpful both for you as well as the doctors. It can be made in the following format:

Name: _____   Age: _____

S.No.	Name of the medicine	Dose	Target symptoms	Date started	Benefits/ Side effects	Date stopped, Reason

Medication Chart

Important papers to be kept in the insurance file

1. Insurance policy
2. Insurance premium receipts
3. Doctor's fee receipts
4. Diagnostic test's receipts
5. Medicine bills

While medicines will help to reduce the symptoms, early intervention will help the child to learn the basic life skills followed by academic skills. The next chapter addresses early intervention and education.

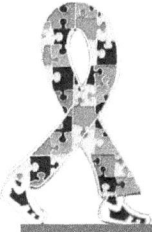

Chapter 11

Early Intervention and Education

Early intervention is a system of services that helps infants and toddlers having developmental delays and disabilities. There are no medications which can cure ASD but research has shown that early intervention during the toddler years can significantly improve a child's development. While early intervention is extremely important but intervention at a later stage is also useful.

Some of the common features of effective early intervention programmes as observed by the American Academy of Pediatrics include the following:

1. Starting early i.e. as soon as a child is diagnosed with ASD.
2. Having one on one time with the therapist.
3. Providing focused learning activities for at least 25 hours per week every month.
4. Organizing educational and training programmes for the parents and family.
5. Providing structured, routine and visual cues to reduce distractions.
6. Recording the child's progress at regular intervals and adjusting it according to the needs of the child.
7. Proper guidance to the child in using the learned skills in new environment.

While searching for a school, parents can select it on the basis of the above criteria.

Before selecting the appropriate treatment plan for the child the therapist assesses the child by filling a questionnaire. This is done by observing the child and taking the help of the parents.

Some of the sample questions are:

Social

1. Does the child make eye contact? _____

2. How does the child respond to a hug from parent? _____

3. How does the child respond to a new toy? _____

Communication
1. Does the child have speech? _____
2. How does the child communicate? Does he/she prefer any of the following methods? _____
   a. Gesture
   b. Body language
   c. Eye gaze
   d. Touching the object
3. Can the child follow directions? _____

Behaviour
1. Does the child display emotions appropriate to the situation? _____

2. How does the child display the following emotions? _____

   a. Happiness
   b. Anger
   c. Fear
   d. Pain
3. Which of the following behaviours are displayed by the child? _____

   a. Hyperactivity
   b. Repetitive behaviour
   c. Screaming
   d. Unawareness of danger

Apart from the questionnaire the therapist uses the following intelligence scales for proper planning:

   a. WISC (Wechsler Intelligence Scale for Children) – Verbal and Non Verbal intellectual ability
   b. LIPS (Leiter International Performance Scale) – Totally non verbal

There are several models of treatment. Some of them are:

1. Treatment and Education of Autistic and related Communication handicapped Children (TEACCH)
2. Developmental, Individual difference, Relationship (DIR)
3. Interpersonal Synchrony

No treatment is a perfect treatment. Moreover a particular treatment might be beneficial for a particular child while the same treatment might not be effective for the other child with the same diagnosis.

The curriculum should generally focus on the following:

a. Independently doing the daily living skills like brushing, eating, changing clothes etc.
b. Reduce aggressive and inappropriate behaviours like stimming, pica etc.
c. Developing social skills like eye contact, greeting etc.
d. Developing communication.

One of the commonly beneficial treatments is Applied Behaviour Analysis (ABA).

Applied Behaviour Analysis (ABA)

Behaviour
Behaviour is anything a person says or does. In other words, behaviour is the range of actions or mannerisms made by an organism. All behaviour is communicative. It serves a function. More than one behaviour may serve the same function, for example, in order to avoid something a child may scream, cry, put his/her head down or throw things. On the other hand, one behaviour may have several functions, for example by biting, a child may express his/her fear or anxiety or frustration of not able to tell what he/she wants.

Functions of behaviour
Any behaviour serves one of the following functions:

1. Escaping or avoiding a situation or a task.
2. Obtaining a desired object or a result.
3. Trying to get self satisfaction, feel good, self calm.
4. Getting other people's attention (This could be both positive or negative).
5. Attempt to get control over the immediate environment.

ABC's of Behaviour
Antecedent – The events, stimulus, environment, circumstances or situations that precede a behaviour is known as antecedent.

Behaviour – The speech or action of the child is known as behaviour.

Consequence – The events that happen to the child immediately after a particular behaviour is known as consequence.

The therapist makes a chart based on ABC for evaluation and treatment. For example,

Date	Antecedent	Behaviour	Consequence	Remedial Action
14/7/14	The therapist asks the child to sit on a chair.	The child hits the therapist.	The therapist takes the child to a different room.	The therapist asks the child to sit on a cushion or a bean bag.

Iceberg Model of Behaviour

Physically aggressive behaviour is generally caused by anxiety due to some underlying problems. This behaviour can be compared to an iceberg.

An iceberg is a large piece of ice that has been broken off from a glacier and floats in the ocean. It is difficult to judge its depth from a distance. In 1912, the great ship Titanic collided with an iceberg and lost the lives of 1500 passengers.

Similarly, we can only see the tip of the iceberg when we see an aggressive behaviour of the child. The underlying problems could be his/her sensory overload, social interaction problem, communication problem, stress and frustration due to his/her inability. So in the example given above by hitting the therapist the child is trying to draw the attention of the therapist in order to communicate his/her discomfort.

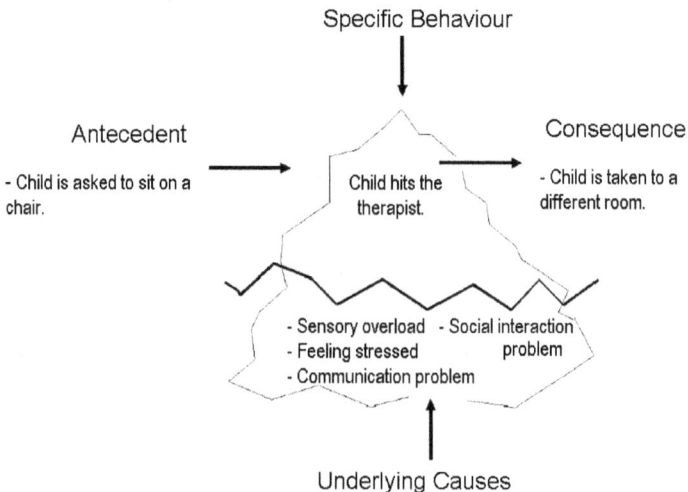

Iceberg Model of Behaviour

Autism – A Handbook of Diagnosis & Treatment of ASD

What is ABA?

Applied behaviour analysis is a systematic way of observing someone's behaviour, identifying desirable changes in the behaviour and then applying various principles and techniques to bring positive and observable change in the behaviour. It is based on operant conditioning theory which says that the behaviour of a person changes as a consequence of the punishment or reward which they receive after a particular behaviour.

Applied behaviour analysis has seven dimensions

1. Analytic
2. Applied
3. Behavioural
4. Effective
5. Generalized
6. Systematic
7. Technical

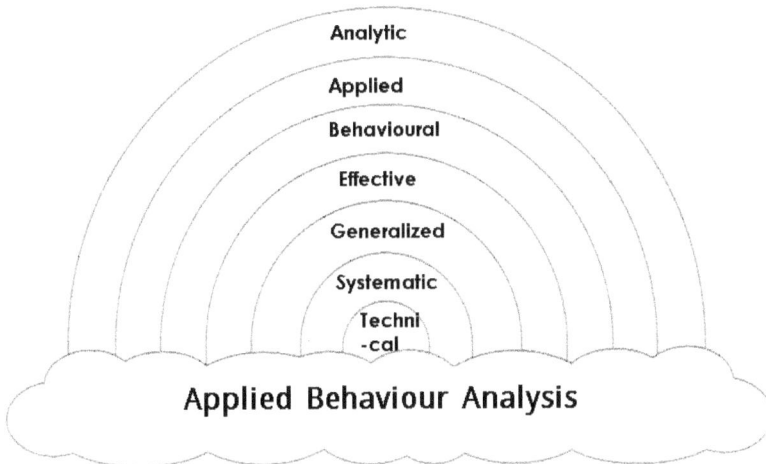

The seven dimensions of ABA

Basic Principles of ABA

The basic principles of ABA are Reinforcement, Shaping, Prompting, Chaining, Punishment, Extinction and Discrete trial training.

1. Reinforcement

Every human being feels motivated to do pleasurable activities while they try to avoid the unpleasant ones.

Reinforcement is a process which increases the likelihood of a positive behaviour to recur by using any activity, event, condition or an environment. Reinforcement strengthens the behaviour. Depending on the child's liking the reinforcement can be given in the edible form or sensory form.

Types of Reinforcement

a. **Positive reinforcement –** The addition of a stimulus to increase a certain behaviour is known as positive reinforcement. For example, when a child stops hitting or throwing things (desired behaviour) a lollipop is given (adding stiumulus).

b. **Negative reinforcement –** The taking away of a stimulus to increase a certain behaviour. For example a child stops screaming (desired behaviour) when the music is switched off (stimulus taken away).

2. Shaping

This technique gradually teaches new behaviour. It is achieved by reinforcing successive approximations or small steps of the target behaviour. For example, to teach a child how to wash hands the process is broken into number of steps and each step is taught independently.

Serial number	A	B
1.	Dirty hands	Go near the wash basin
2.	Wash basin	Open the tap
3.	Open the tap	Wet your hands
4.	Wet hands	Pick up the soap
5.	Pick up the soap	Rub it on your hand
6.	Rub the soap on hand	Keep the soap back on soap dish
7.	Soap foam on hand	Wash your hands
8.	Washed hands	Turn off the tap
9.	Clean and wet hands	Dry your hands using a towel

3. Prompting

This technique provides a cue or a hint to increase the probability of a correct response.

Types of Prompt

a. **Verbal Prompt** – In this type of prompt verbal cues are given in a simple language (which the child understands) to follow direction and respond correctly. For example, in the second step of the hand washing example, after the child reaches near the wash basin the verbal prompt open is given, then the child knows he/she has to open the tap.

b. **Physical Prompt** – In physical prompt, physical guidance is provided to students to perform a particular skill. In this case to perform the second step the child's hand is put on the tap. So the child knows he/she has to open it.

c. **Visual Prompt** – This includes the use of pictures, gesture, demonstration or modeling to help the students. This technique is useful for those children who have difficulty in understanding a language. In this case pictures are made for each step and shown to the child to follow.

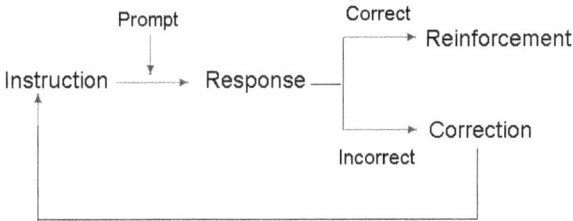

Arrow diagram of prompt

d. **Fading Prompts** – The process of systematically withdrawing prompts and still getting the desired result is known as fading. Fading is generally performance based and not time based. Verbal prompts are hard to fade whereas physical prompts are comparatively easy to fade.

4. Chaining

The process of breaking down of a complicated task into responses that are linked to one another is known as chaining of behaviour.

Types of Chaining

a. **Forward Chaining** – Each step is mastered by the student before the next step of skill is added in the forward direction. In the hand washing example the child is reinforced when he/she is able to do the first step on his/her own. Remaining steps are done with the help of the therapist. Next time the child is reinforced when he/she can do the first two steps. Gradually the steps are increased for getting a reinforcement till the target behaviour is achieved.

b. **Backward Chaining** – In this the last step is taught first and then each step is added in the backward direction. In this case step 8 will be taught first in the hand washing example.

c. **Total task Presentation** – In this the student performs all the steps in a sequence until all the steps are mastered. In this case all the eight steps are taught everyday till the child masters it.

5. Punishment

Contingent presentation of a stimulus (something which the student dislikes), immediately following a response (student's inappropriate behaviour) which decreases the future probability of the same response is known as punishment.

Types of Punishment

According to psychologist B.F Skinner there are two types of punishment.

a. **Positive Punishment –** The punishment which involves presenting an aversive stimulus after a behaviour has occurred is known as positive punishment. This is also known as *"punishment by application"*. For example, asking the child to sit at a place which he/she doesn't like.

b. **Negative Punishment** - The punishment which involves taking away a desirable stimulus after a behaviour has occurred is known as negative punishment. This is also known as *"punishment by removal"*. For example, taking away the favourite toy or taking away the feel good cloth.

6. Extinction

The process of reducing undesirable behaviour by withholding the positive reinforcer that maintains the undesirable behaviour is known as extinction.

Effectiveness of Punishment and Extinction

There is a controversy regarding the effectiveness of punishment and extinction in decreasing undesirable behaviour. Some psychologists feel that both these strategies produce a temporary change in the behaviour. Some feel that they have an adverse effect on the behaviour since child can have an unintended consequence. He/she may withdraw himself/herself or develop a tolerance to punishment or develop unnecessary fear. The child might even become more aggressive.

7. Discrete Trial Training

This is an instructional approach in which a series of distinct, repeated lessons are taught along with reinforcement of the learned behaviour till the new behaviour becomes a habit.

The following flow chart can be used to make a study plan for a child.

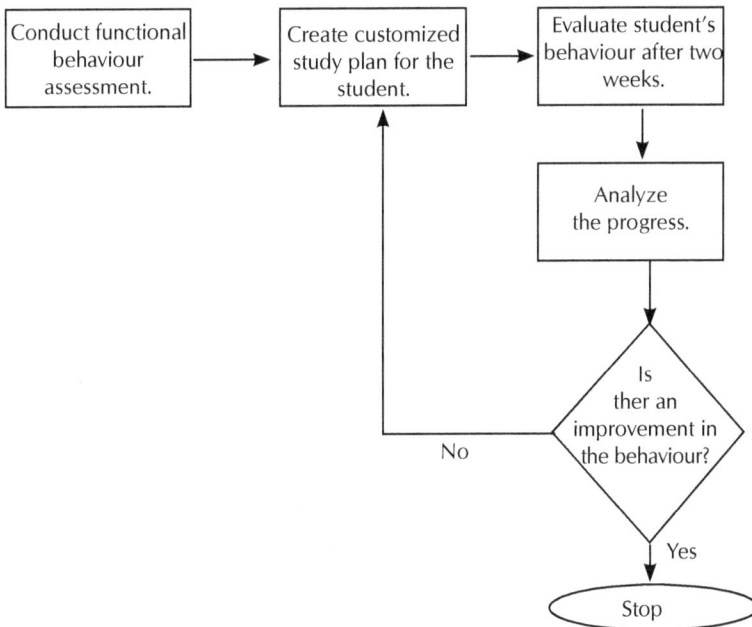

Flowchart of study plan

A.I.I.M.S uses the following approach after the diagnosis of autism.

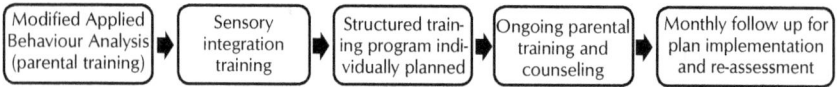

| Modified Applied Behaviour Analysis (parental training) | → | Sensory integration training | → | Structured training program individually planned | → | Ongoing parental training and counseling | → | Monthly follow up for plan implementation and re-assessment |

A common question comes to the mind of every parent – "Should we send the child to mainstream schools or special schools? What will people say if we send him/her to a special school?" No doubt the negative comments of people around us hurt but our main aim is to improve the child and not to improve the comments of the people.

In my opinion greater improvement will take place in our little prince/princesses if they are sent to special schools since the teachers there are specially trained.

Some of the drawbacks of sending special needs children to mainstream school are:

1. The mainstream schools do not have the infrastructure to handle autism.
2. The teachers do not have the special training. Hence they might scold the special need child unnecessarily.
3. The speed of teaching might be an information overload for the special need children.
4. The special need children often have the need to learn the basic life skills first before entering into academic learning which might not be taken care of in mainstream schools.
5. The mainstream schools have a fixed syllabus for all the students whereas in special schools there is an individualized education plan for every student.
6. Due to the large number of students in a class the teachers are not able to give individual attention.
7. Due to the lack of awareness of autism the classmates may bully the special need child.
8. The parents of typical children might criticize the special need child in front of his/her parent.
9. The unsuitable teaching method may decrease the self esteem and self confidence of the special need child which may further lead to regression.

10. The child may need help in eating and drinking even at an older age which is not provided in the mainstream schools.

I have listed many schools in different states and union territories in Chapter 26. My humble request to the parents is to go through the list and do some research work if there are better schools near their residence and send their ward to one of the schools specially designed for autistic children.

After the childhood comes the development of adolescent years. Parents should start preparing their children for adolescence from their tween age (the age from 10 to 12 years i.e. between childhood and adolescent).

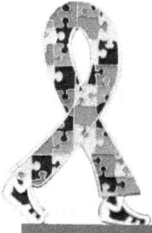

Chapter 12

Adolescent Years

Adolescence is defined as the period in human development that occurs between the beginning of puberty and adulthood. It is also termed as teenage. A lot of hormonal changes occur within the body which results in physical as well as psychological changes. Children with autism go through the same hormonal changes as the typical children undergo during their teenage. The only difference is that they may react differently due to their lack of communication and social skills. This is a difficult time for both children (typical or non typical) and parents.

Once a parent told me that her daughter's autism was getting worse after twelve years. I immediately pointed out autism was not getting worse but her daughter was entering adolescence. As a parent or teacher or therapist we should be aware of teenage behaviours in order to tackle them properly.

Expected teenage behaviours in children with autism

1. The irritability may increase.
2. They tend to become moody and arrogant.
3. They may become more non communicative.
4. The attention span may decrease.
5. They may insist more on sameness and orderliness.
6. There might be an onset of seizure, those who had seizures in their childhood may develop it again during teen years.

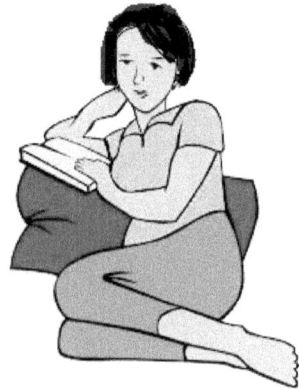

Sad teenager

7. Physical changes like underarm hair, pubic hair and maturation of reproductive organs may cause distress.

8. During teenage most of the children develop the awareness that they are different. This may add to the distress in some children.
9. Anxiety and stress may increase leading to depression. Girls might be more stressed due to the start of menstruation (periods).
10. They may develop an interest towards the opposite sex.
11. They may develop a tendency to masturbate.
12. Echolalia, stimming and self injurious behaviour might increase in

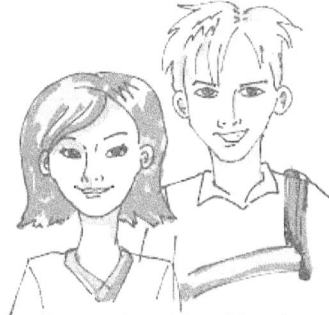

Boy and a girl as friends during adolescent years

some children while it may app-ear for the first time in others.
13. They (specially girls) are more vulnerable to sexual abuse. The attraction towards the opposite sex is natural at this age but their one innocent inappropriate physical or verbal gesture might put them into serious trouble.

Autism as a blessing during teenage

1. There is no peer pressure.
2. Children with autism normally do not have a demanding nature during teenage. For example, they do not insist on buying all the latest electronic gadgets like iPhone, iPad etc.
3. During teenage most of the children develop the awareness that they are different. In some children this motivates them to learn the social skills, communication skills and interact with peer group. They develop the feeling of belonging. Taking the advantage of the situation children with ASD can be sent to normal activity schools (music, art etc.) and allowed to mix with typically growing adolescents.

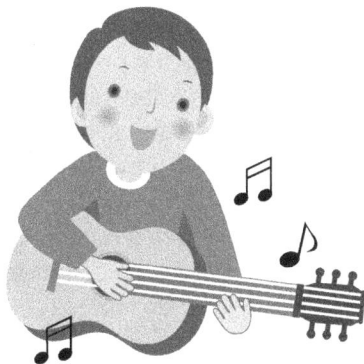

Teenage boy playing guitar

4. They tend to develop special interests. This should be encouraged.

5. Generally they do not tend to develop the bad habit of smoking, drinking etc.

Good news

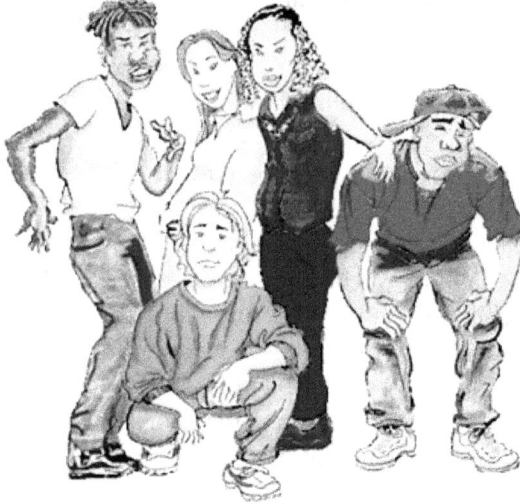

A group of teenagers

Various research study has found that those children who had early intervention showed a remarkable improvement during teen years. Although the result varies from study to study but on an average there is an improvement in 40-80% cases.

Guidelines for parents

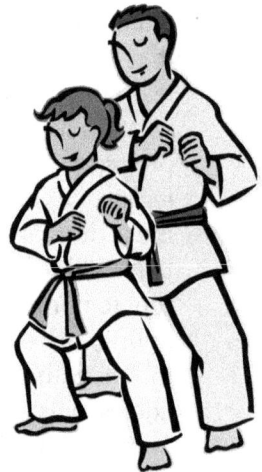

1. Parents need to make positive behaviour plans. The adolescents need to be taught about personal hygiene and self care skills. They need to be taught about the private body parts, appropriate and inappropriate sexual behaviour.

2. Encourage and increase the physical activity of the adolescent. They find difficulty in team sports. So individual sports like badminton, swimming, karate etc. can be encouraged.

Father and teenager doing karate

3. Adolescents undergo a rapid growth during their teen years. They increase both in height and weight. Due to this growth spurt the nutritional needs are also high. Parents need to take care of that.

4. Need to plan for medical transition from pediatrician to a general physician who is efficient in treating autism. Sometimes it becomes difficult to understand whether an aggressive behaviour signifies normal adolescence or some other underlying physical problem. At that time a general medical check up might prove to be useful.

5. In case of seizure or depression some medicine might be required. If the child is already having a medicine there might be a need to increase the dose with doctor's consultation. The girls might need some medicine for menstrual cramps.

6. Parents need to make their children aware of the physical changes of adolescence by eleven or twelve years of age. The girls need to be aware of developing mammary glands and menstruation. Pictures, videos etc. can be used for the explanation.

Irrespective of childhood, tween or adolescence, parents are always concerned about the safety of their children. Some of the safety tips are given in the next chapter for a quick reference.

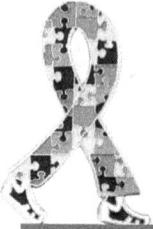

Chapter 13

Safety Tips

Child safety is a significant concern for all parents. The occasional cut, bruise, fall or even fracture is a part of growing up. This is normal for all children but children with ASD have an increased risk of accidents and injuries. Hence, parents need to be extra careful.

Some safety tips

Around the house

1. Cover the exposed electrical outlets and extension cords.
2. Try not to use table fans (Prefer ceiling fans).
3. Safeguard the electrical appliances like washing machine, microwave, electric iron etc.
4. Keep the cleaning supplies like bleach, phenyl, laundry detergents etc. under lock and key.
5. Keep hazardous substances under lock and key. This includes insect repellants and poisons, fertilizers, paints, brake fluid, kerosene oil, correction fluid etc. as well as the combustible substances like match box, gas lighter etc.
6. Keep the medicines out of the reach of the child (Even a regular medicine of the child can be harmful if taken in over dose).
7. Keep sharp objects like knife, scissors etc. out of the reach of the child.
8. Do not use glass furniture. Make sure that the edges of the furniture are not sharp.
9. Avoid hanging glass photo frames.
10. Keep your child's pediatrician's telephone number handy.
11. Be careful about the plants which you grow in your garden. Some of the commonly grown household plants like dumb cane, caladium, oleander etc. are very poisonous.

Poisonous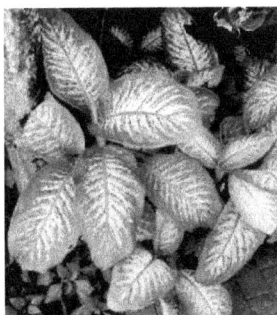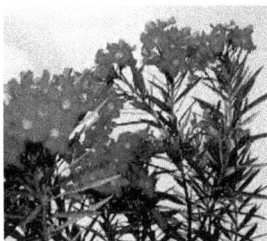

plants

household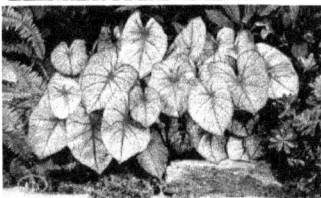

Some common poisonous household plants

Outside the house

Some children with ASD have the tendency to wander around. They do not understand the concept of any danger. Hence, the entrance/exit door of the house should be locked properly all the time. Even when the parents take their child out they should be careful. The following type of identity card may be attached to the dress of the child while going out.

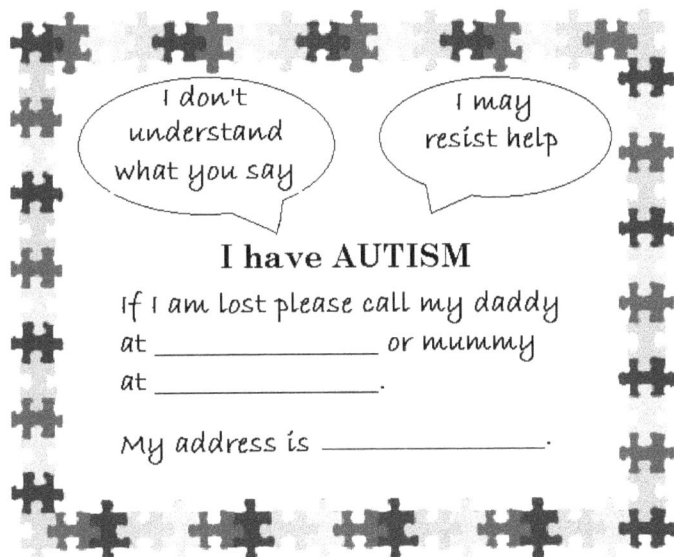

Identity card for a child

In spite of taking precautions it is not possible to prevent all injuries. Be prepared to handle it efficiently. If possible do a course on first aid or else read a book on first aid and keep a first aid kit ready at home.

You can prevent injuries to a great extent if you better understand your child's sensory issues.

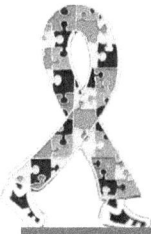

Chapter 14

Managing Sensory Issues

Sense Organs

The five basic human sensory organs are eye, ear, nose, tongue and skin. These organs have nerve endings which take in information from the surrounding and carry them to the brain so that the body can act on it. Without sensory organs we would not be able to make any sense of our surroundings or environment. The senses related to the various organs are: *vision, olfactory, auditory, tactile and gustatory.*

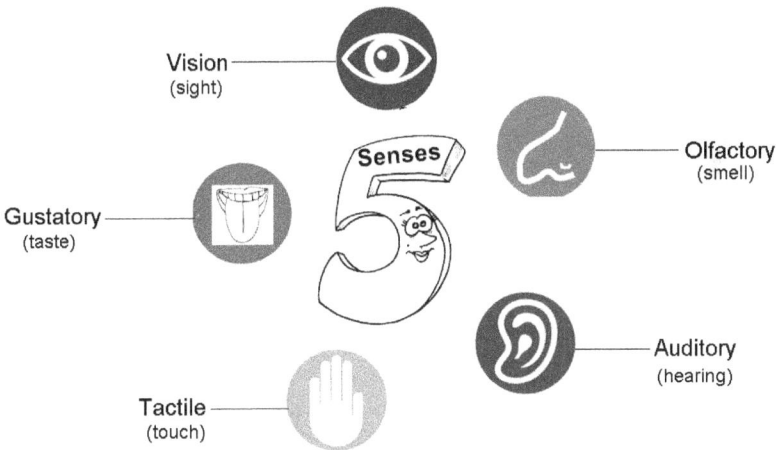

Vision
(sight)

Senses

Olfactory
(smell)

Gustatory
(taste)

Tactile
(touch)

Auditory
(hearing)

Five basic sense organs of human being

Some other senses are *vestibular, proprioception, thermoception, nociception* and *chronoception*. The organs responsible for these senses are inner ear, joints as well as muscles, skin and brain.

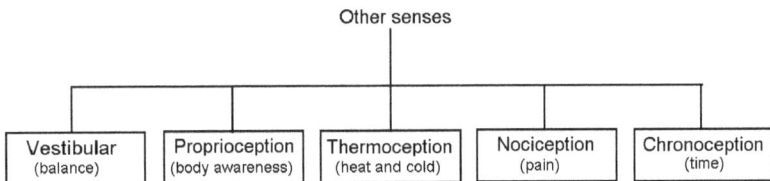

Other senses

| Vestibular (balance) | Proprioception (body awareness) | Thermoception (heat and cold) | Nociception (pain) | Chronoception (time) |

Other sense organs of human being

Sensory perception in autism

Children with autism often experience the senses in a different manner. This means that they perceive the world differently. Some of them are hypersensitive while others are hyposensitive. The result of these sensitivities is often seen in their behaviour.

Hypersensitivity –When a child's sensitivity is high or when a child is over sensitive to stimuli it is known as hypersensitivity.

Hyposensitivity –When a child's sensitivity is low or when a child is under sensitive to stimuli it is known as hyposensitivity.

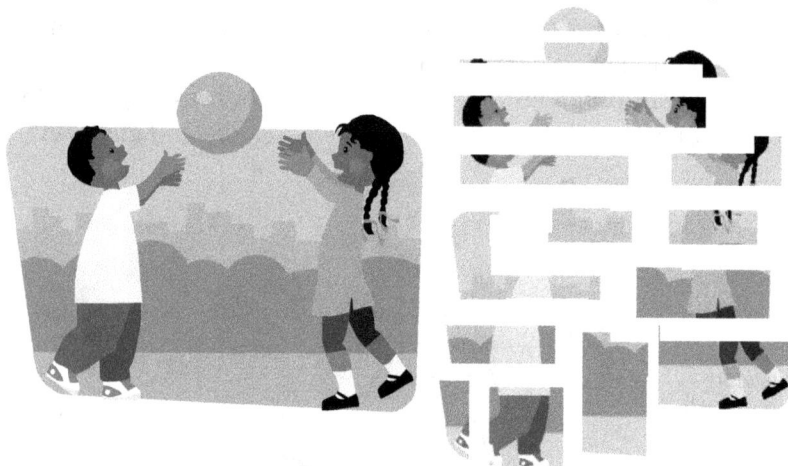

The picture on the left may appear as fragmented (right picture) to some children with ASD.

Let us look at some of the perceptions of an autistic individual. (See the table)

Sense organ	Sense	Perception
Eye	Vision (sight)	*Hypersensitive* (Avoider) • Overwhelmed by bright light. • A central object may appear magnified but things on the periphery may be blurred. • Central vision may be blurred but peripheral vision quite sharp. • Poor depth perception – problems with catching and throwing. *Hyposensitive* (Seeker) • May have difficulty in tracking moving things. • Images may appear fragmented and distorted. • Individuals may focus on small things but miss out big things.
Ear	Auditory (hearing)	*Hypersensitive* Moderate noises gets magnified and hence become painful. As a result : • Some children react strongly and may just have a shut down period. • Others may get carried away by the background sound. This often leads to difficulties in concentration. *Hyposensitive* • Normal volume might be too low, hence might prefer loud sound. • Might enjoy crowded, noisy places or bang doors and objects.
Nose	Olfactory (smell)	*Hypersensitive* • Over sensitive to smell. Certain smell may make them feel sick. This may cause toileting problems, dislike certain soaps, creams etc. *Hyposensitive* • Have low smelling power. As a result certain food items might not be appetizing.

Tongue	Gustatory (taste)	*Hypersensitive* • Over active taste buds. Certain food textures may cause discomfort hence try to avoid some kind of food. *Hyposensitive* • Under active taste buds. Can't make any difference in various food types.
Skin	Tactile (touch)	*Hypersensitive* • Certain textures of fabric may feel unusually uncomfortable. It might hurt the skin or be itchy. • May dislike washing and brushing hair since head is sensitive. • A light touch may feel like a heavy blow. • May not like hugs and kisses. *Hyposensitive* • Less sensitivity to touch. • May like tight clothes, play rough games, hit hard on things, etc. • May enjoy tight hugs. • Generally have a high threshold to pain. May self harm.
Inner ear	Vestibular (balance)	*Hypersensitive* • May have difficulty in balancing and movement (up and down, going round in circles etc.). • Generally love flat surfaces. • May get motion sickness. *Hyposensitive* • Love to spin in circles. • Prefers to be on the move all the time, finds it difficult to sit still.

Muscles and joints	Proprioception (body awareness)	Hypersensitive
		• Difficulty with fine motor skills like tying shoe lace, buttoning the shirt etc.
		• Moves whole body to look at something.
		• May lean against wall or furniture.
		• May avoid big groups.
		Hyposensitive
		Lacks coordination in body movement. As a result:
		• May stand too close to people.
		• May bump into people.
		• May bump into furniture.
		• May like to jump.

In order to help the child the first step for the parents would be to identify the sensory problem. Next step would be to find a fun way of satisfying the sensory need. There are different ways by which we can satisfy the sensory need of the child.

Management of some sensory issues

Vision problem: Bright light hurt.

Possible solution: Use low power LED lights. Use sunglass. Sunglass can be used even at night if required.

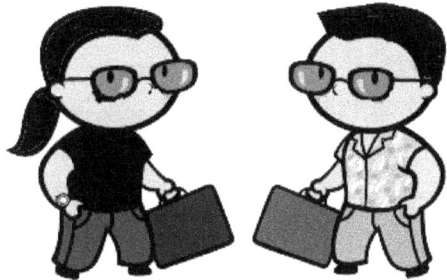
Teenagers wearing sunglass

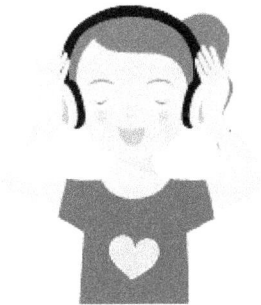
Girl wearing headphone

Auditory problem: Normal sound appears to be loud.

Possible solution: Use ear plug or head phone.

Olfactory problem: Smell of soap, oil, shampoo, household cooking etc. creates problem.

Possible solution: Try lavender or sandalwood soap. Light lavender or sandalwood incense sticks or candles while cooking.

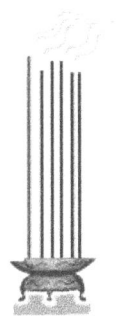
Lavender incense sticks

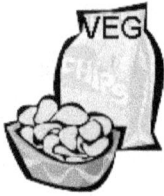

Vegetable chips

Gustatory problem: Pica the problem of licking or chewing non edible items.

Possible solution: Try sugarless chewing gum. Try fat free vegetable chips.

Tactile problem: Hits hard on things.

Possible solution: Try weighted blanket. (Stuff the blanket with sand for giving weight).

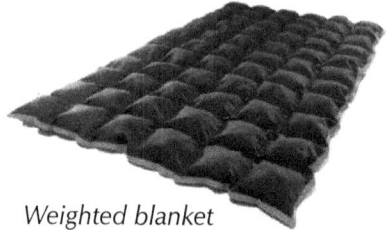

Weighted blanket

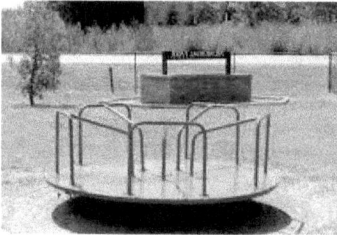

Merry go round

Vestibular problem: Spins in circle.

Possible solution: Take the child to the park on merry go round.

Proprioception problem: Motor development problem.

Possible solution: Try spike balls, plastacine, yo-yo, yoga ball. Yoga ball also improves the blood circulation.

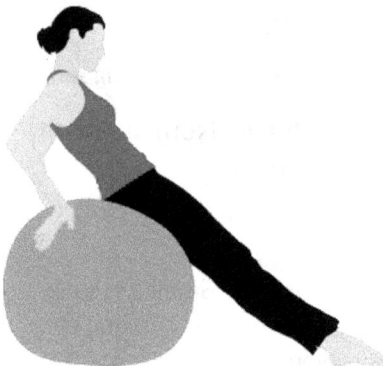

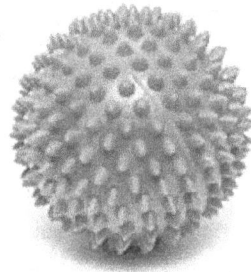

Yoga ball and spike ball

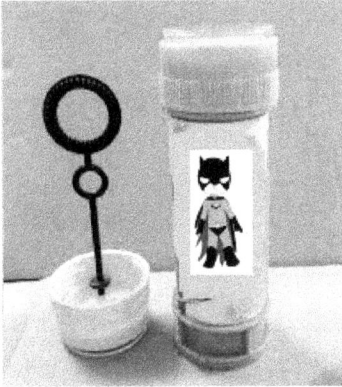

Bubble toy and pinwheel

For various neuromuscular developments use colourful balloons, mouth organ, soap bubble toy, pinwheel, beanbag chair etc.

The lack of satisfaction of sensory need, inability to communicate properly and various health discomforts leads to the behaviour problems in autistic children. Let us see how to deal with the behaviour problems in the next chapter.

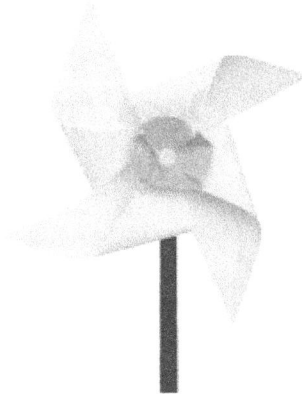

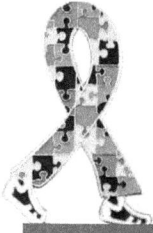

Chapter 15

Dealing with Behaviour Problems

Behaviour is the range of actions and mannerisms made by an individual in relation with himself/herself or his/her environment. Children with autism often exhibit unusual behaviour. For example, they may make strange sounds, talk to themselves, ask the same question again and again, have meltdown, do stimming, etc. There is generally a reason for this kind of behaviour. It can be their own method of coping with a particular situation or it can be their attempt to communicate.

Strange Sounds

Many children in the autistic spectrum have little or no speech at all. Researchers are not sure of the cause. It is possible that the speech centre of the brain does not develop properly. It is even possible that they choose not to speak or to speak less because they find it difficult to understand the meaning of words. Possibly the words appear as strange sounds in their ears. Hence, they try to reproduce it by making strange sounds.

Self talking

Many children have the habit of talking to themselves. This could be due to their unawareness of the presence of other people or it could be due to their lack of social communication skill. Probably they find solace in talking to themselves.

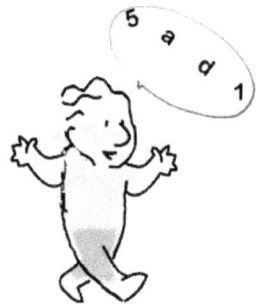

A child talking to himself

Asking the same question

Some children who are able to talk have the habit of asking the same question again and again. This probably indicates their anxious behaviour. They want to feel safe and secured by listening to the same answer again and again. Like mantra chanting, listening to the same answer repeatedly could be comforting for them.

Apart from unusual behaviour autistic children often go through a rage cycle.

Rage Cycle

The children with autism are prone to stress and anxiety which results in a rage cycle. The parents can help to reduce that by trying to manage the stress level of the child.

The rage cycle is a three step process commonly known as 3 R's.

1. Rumbling
2. Rage
3. Recovery

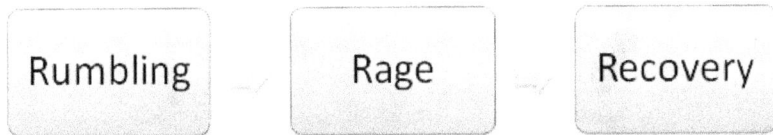

Rumbling — Rage — Recovery

Three stages of rage cycle

Rumbling

This is the pre stage of rage or meltdown and normally happens when children are exposed to triggers. The inner struggle starts within the child and its effect is seen on the behaviour.

Some behaviour which suggests rumbling:

1. Biting nails.
2. Clenching fist.
3. Tapping feet.
4. Tensed muscles.
5. Rocking back and forth.
6. Tearing paper.
7. Making strange sounds or talking at a high pitch.
8. Grinding teeth.
9. Cold or sweaty palm.
10. Heavy breathing.

11. Fast heartbeat.

If the parents can intervene and lower the anxiety at this level it will not reach the rage/meltdown level.

Some strategies to lower rumbling

1. Moving closer to the child. If the child likes to be hugged, giving him/her a hug will be reassuring. If not just by being close to him/her may lessen the stress.
2. Remove the child from the environment which is causing the difficulty. Taking him/her to another room might solve the problem.

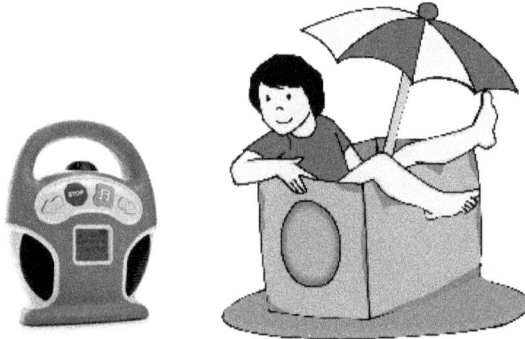

A child trying to relax at his calm down space

3. Sending the child to his/her calm-down space may relax him/her. The calm down space can be some cozy part of the house where the child feels comfortable by spending some time alone. Keep a music player with headphone, sunglass, pillow, cushion and blanket as per the sensory need of the child, water, favourite toy, paper and colours. Arindam's (my friend's son) calm down space is inside a box fitted with comfortable mattress.
4. Going for a short walk with the child helps many times.
5. Diverting the child's attention into something else.
6. Showing his next routine in the form of visual cards may release his/her tension.

Most of the time if rumbling is not controlled it leads to rage or meltdown.

Rage/Meltdown

All children have tantrums and temper tantrums but children

with ASD often have meltdowns which are erratic and very difficult to handle. By definition,

Meltdown is an involuntary increase in temper tantrum like behaviour. It involves screaming, shouting, pushing, biting, throwing objects, kicking people, hurting himself/herself etc. It is usually caused by extreme stress.

There are certain differences between tantrums and meltdowns:

S.No.	Temper tantrum	Meltdown
1.	This is a goal driven, want oriented mechanism.	This is a reactive mechanism.
2.	The child is in control of the situation.	The child is not in control of the situation.
3.	The child is concerned about getting a reaction to his behaviour.	The child is not concerned about getting a reaction to his behaviour.
4.	The child is careful about his/her own safety during temper tantrums.	The child is not bothered about his/her own safety during meltdowns
5.	If the issue is resolved the temper tantrum ends.	Meltdowns are not goal dependent hence they take a long time to get in control.
6.	Temper tantrums tend to fade away after five years of age.	Meltdowns remain upto the adulthood.

Possible causes of meltdown

1. Unexpected and unpredictable situation.
2. Unfamiliar or new situation.
3. Change in daily routine (Even a little change can cause a lot of stress in autistic children).
4. Overstimulation of sense organs or cognitive skills.
5. Emotional or information overload.
6. Task performance demand by parents/ teachers.
7. Repeated interruption of their stereo typed behaviour.

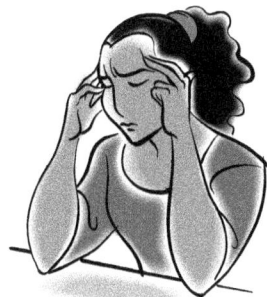

A teenager with a bout of headache

8. Physical discomfort like headache, acidity etc. and the inability to express it to get relief.
9. Failure to understand social situation.

Strategy to get over meltdown

Once the meltdown sets in it usually takes some time before the child settles down. The safety of the child should be the main focus at this stage. If the child allows to touch, a gentle massage may help him/her to calm down. In extreme cases the child needs to be given some nerve relaxant medicine. Scolding or slapping the child will make the situation worse. So don't do that.

Practical tips for parents to reduce meltdowns

1. Maintain a meltdown chart to find the triggers in the following format:

Date and Time	Triggers	Duration of meltdown	Steps taken to subside the meltdown

Try to avoid potential triggers as far as possible.
2. Take care of sensory issues. For example, make the child wear sunglasses even at night if you are going out at night especially during festival time and the decoration lights bother the child.
3. Do the HATS test from time to time. HATS stands for
   - **H**ungry
   - **A**ngry
   - **T**hirsty/Tired
   - **S**tressed
4. Make visual cards for the child for all activities (Refer the next chapter).
5. Prepare the child in advance in case there is going to be any change of routine.
6. Use transition tools. For example, a picture card like the following will convey that the child will be playing after he/she finishes milk so that he/she is mentally prepared for the next activity.

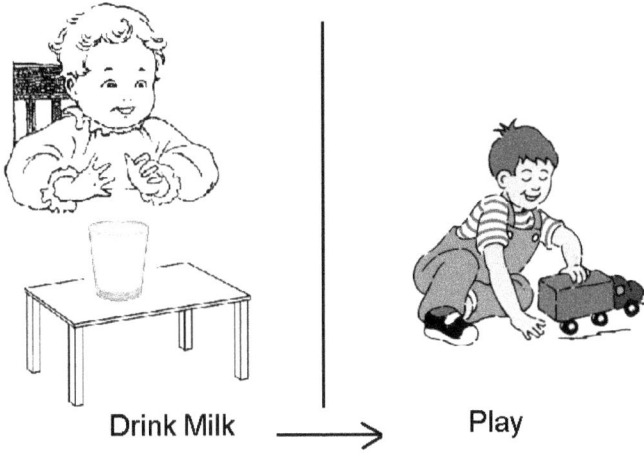

Drink Milk ⟶ Play

Picture cards to show transition of activity

Recovery

This is the post stage of meltdown. The child may not fully remember what all happened during meltdown. It is better to give some rest to the child and make him/her do the activities he/she enjoys and then follow his usual routine.

Coping tips for parents

Even after the child settles down the parents feel upset about the situation. There are no services to match the needs of the parents in our country. Although there are no easy answers to this but some of the following coping methods might help.

Coping methods for parents

1. Cease what you were doing that did not work.
2. Consciously choose to have positive feelings. The rage was not your fault. It was due to a situation and not due to you.
3. Control your frustration and try to calm down.
4. Count your blessings.
5. Concentrate on your breathing.

You will be surprised to discover your own inner strength which already exists. I can understand you are thinking it is easier said than done but believe me one of the trusted method is to recite "Gayatri mantra". This mantra is one of the most powerful mantra of Hinduism.

Gayatri Mantra

"Om Bhur Bhuvaha Svaha
Tat Savitur Varenyam
Bhargo Devasya Dhemahi
Dhiyo Yonah Prachodayat."

Meaning of Gayatri Mantra

O God! You are omnipresent and omnipotent. You are the light, knowledge and bliss. You are destroyer of fear and the creator of this universe; you are the greatest of all. We bow and meditate upon your light. May you guide our intellect in the right direction.

Benefits of Gayatri Mantra

Prolonged repetition of this mantra has a beneficial effect both on our body and mind. Some of them are:

1) It protects us from danger.
2) It gives us mental strength.
3) It removes the obstacles from life.
4) It increases our tolerance level.
5) It improves our immune system.
6) It calms our mind.

Another common behaviour problem observed in children with ASD is stimming.

Stimming

An intense repetitive, purposeless body movement is known as stimming. It is a self stimulating behaviour. Psychiatrists use the term "stereotyped behaviour" for stimming. Most of the stimming actions are involuntary in the beginning. Probably it forms a habit later on.

Some examples of stimming:

Sr. No.	Sense	Stimulatory action
1.	Visual(sight)	• Staring at patterns • Dangling objects in front of the eye. • Lining up objects in a definite order. • Staring at light or fan. • Turning light switches on and off repeatedly.

2.	Auditory(hearing)	• Making deep vocal sounds or high pitched shrieking. • Tapping fingers. • Grinding teeth. • Repeating portions of songs at inappropriate time.
3.	Olfactory(smell)	• Rubbing all kinds of objects on the nose. • Smelling other people. • Smelling objects. • Putting fingers or other objects inside the nose.
4.	Gustatory(taste)	• Licking different objects (non edible). • Putting different objects inside the mouth. • Rubbing different objects on lips, teeth, chin etc. • Licking body parts.
5.	Tactile(touch)	• Rubbing a particular type of cloth or a particular object on the body. • Walking on toes. • Scratching.
6.	Vestibular (balance)	• Rocking back and forth. • Spinning or twirling. • Banging head against the wall. • Walking on toes. • Hand flapping.
7.	Proprioception (body awareness)	• Jumping. • Lying on the floor and irregular movement of legs.

Possible causes of stimming

1. Provides sensory stimulation.
2. Reduces anxiety which is a common problem in children with ASD.

3. Reduction in physical pain. For example, banging head might give a relief to the headache.
4. Expression of excitement or pent up emotions.
5. Self soothing and calming.

Should stimming be stopped?

This is a controversial question. Some doctors say parents should try to stop it since most of the stimming actions are harmful and socially unacceptable. Others believe that if stimming is totally stopped then frequency of meltdown will increase. In my opinion parents should allow the stimming actions which are not harmful for example, arranging objects in a definite order and try to reduce the other stimming by replacement behaviour, for example, licking objects can be replaced by giving a lollipop.

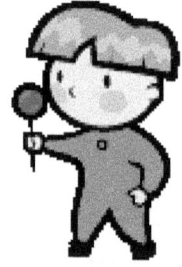

A boy given lollipop to lick

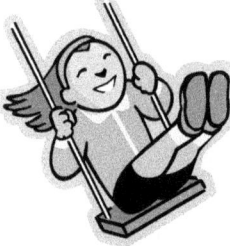

Replacement behaviour

An alternative behaviour which can replace an undesirable behaviour is known as a replacement behaviour.

Rocking back and forth replaced by swinging

The following flowchart gives an example of a replacement behaviour.

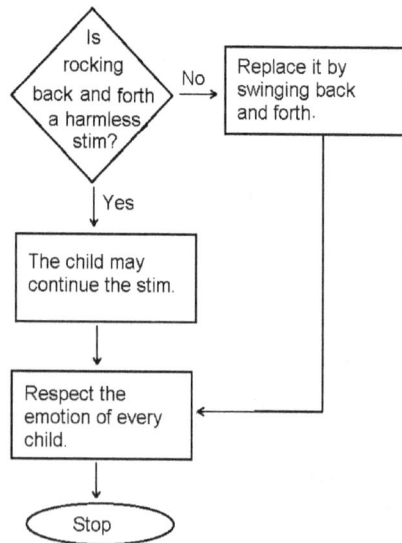

```
        ╱ Is  ╲
       ╱rocking ╲   No    ┌──────────────┐
      ╱back and  ╲───────▶│ Replace it by│
      ╲forth     ╱        │ swinging back│
       ╲a harmless        │ and forth.   │
        ╲stim?╱           └──────────────┘
           │                      │
           │ Yes                  │
           ▼                      │
   ┌──────────────┐               │
   │ The child may│               │
   │ continue the stim.│          │
   └──────────────┘               │
           │                      │
           ▼                      │
   ┌──────────────┐               │
   │ Respect the  │◀──────────────┘
   │ emotion of every│
   │ child.       │
   └──────────────┘
           │
           ▼
        ╭────────╮
        │  Stop  │
        ╰────────╯
```

Flow chart to show a replacement behaviour

Some replacement behaviours

1. If a child is verbal and makes sounds for stimming the child can be put into drama class or music class with emphasis on voice modulation.
2. If a child likes to walk on toes he/she can be put into a dance class specially ballet (if available).
3. If a child repeatedly taps his/her fingers, tabla or drum or keyboard classes can be arranged for him/her.
4. If a child likes to hit things give him/her a squeeze ball or punching bag.
5. If a child finds normal chair too hard make him/her sit on a bean bag.

Admitting a child in an activity class does not necessarily mean that the child has to learn it perfectly but even if the child benefits a little bit it is a big achievement for him/her as well as the parents.

One of the possible causes of undesirable behaviour is lack of good sleep. If sleep problems are resolved there will be lesser chance of rage cycle or stimming.

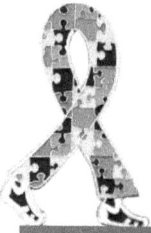

Chapter 16

Managing Sleep

Every living organism needs sleep. The sleep wake cycle known as circadian rhythm is regulated by the light and darkness in the environment of the organism. In humans, this rhythm begins to develop when the child is around six weeks old; by about six months generally all children have a regular sleep wake cycle.

Sleep is necessary to restore our body and mind. It plays a vital role in physical as well as emotional well being of a person. Sleep deprivation (lack of sleep) not only makes a child tired, irritated and sick but also affects his/her learning process during day.

According to the research about 40-80% children with ASD have sleeping problem. Sleep problem can be of different types:

1. Falling asleep
2. Staying asleep
3. Restless sleep
4. Insufficient sleep
5. Irregular sleep wake cycle

There could be different reasons for not getting a restful sleep.

Possible causes of sleep problems

a. Lack of communication

Children with ASD find it hard to comm-unicate what is bothering them. For example, the texture of the bed sheet or the pillow cover might be uncomfortable for them or they might be thirsty at night. Inability to communicate causes helplessness and frustration which affect their sleep.

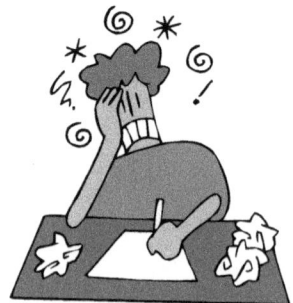

Frustrated teenager

This in turn causes behavioural prob-lems, tiredness, stress, anxiety etc. which further causes difficulty in sleep. Thus it becomes a vicious cycle for them.

b. Side effect of medicines

Due to side effect of some medicine the child might be having some physical discomfort like aches and pains which keeps him/her awake.

c. Environmental factor

Since the sensory perception of these children are different some environmental factors like the room temperature, street light entering the bedroom, hardness of the bed mattress etc. might cause interference with their sleep.

d. Nocturnal Enuresis (Nighttime bedwetting)

Nocturnal enuresis is a common problem in many typically growing children as well as autistic children. This problem generally improves as the children grow older. Normally during adolescence with the change of hormones the problem gets cured automatically. Prior to that you may restrict the fluid intake in the evening, use diaper and take the child to the toilet once or twice during night.

e. Nightmare

Sometimes children wake up due to nightmares. If the child is verbal he/she can express it but if he/she is non verbal then he/she becomes more anxious. Just try to reassure the child that nightmares don't happen in reality. Try to soothe the child in whatever method he/she feels comfortable.

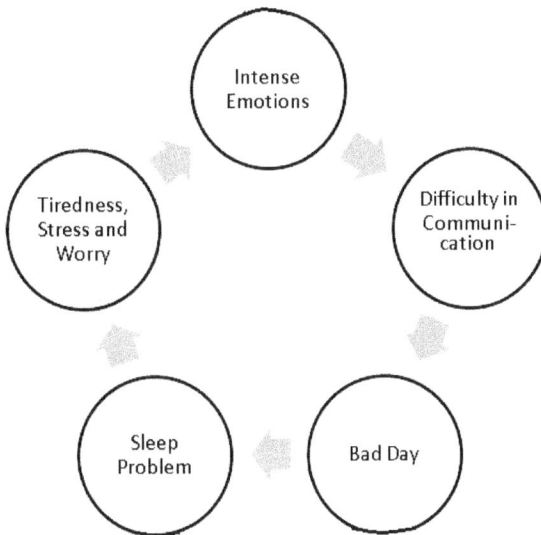

Intense Emotions

Tiredness, Stress and Worry

Difficulty in Communication

Sleep Problem

Bad Day

Vicious cycle of sleep problems

Inability to communicate the intense emotions results in a bad day which further leads to stress and anxiety causing sleep problems.

Some tips to solve sleep problem

a. Make sure that the child gets enough physical exercise during day time on a regular basis.

b. Avoid day time sleep.

c. Eliminate or reduce caffeine containing food and drinks. For example tea, coffee, coke, chocolate etc.

d. Eliminate stimulating activities in the evening.

e. Avoid T.V, computer or video games before bed time. Instead switch on some soothing music.

f. Make the bedroom comfortable for the child. For example, the room temperature, texture of bedsheet /pillow cover which is comfortable for you might not be comfortable for the child. Take care of that.

g. Ensure that the texture of the night dress is comfortable for the child.

h. A gentle massage might help some children.

i. A soothing smell as per the liking of the child is useful.

j. Follow a fixed routine everyday.

k. Make visual aid for the child explaining the bed time routine.

(see the figure)

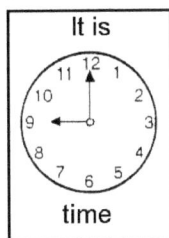

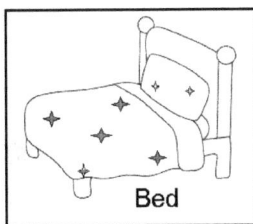

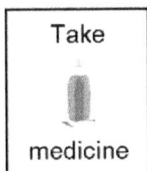

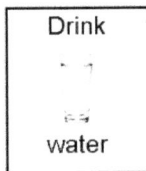

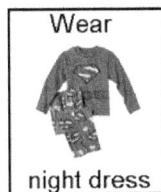

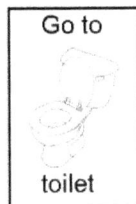

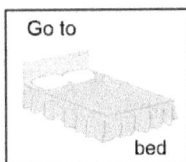

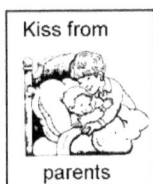

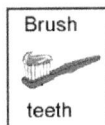

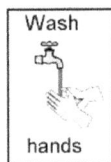

Picture cards for bed time routine

Child's sleep problem often leads to parent's insufficient sleep which adds to their stress and fatigue. Parents should never accept sleep problems to be an inevitable part of autism. Various methods should be tried for helping the child to get a good sleep so that even they get a proper rest at night. Along with sleep regulation another important basic life skill to be taught is toileting skill.

Chapter 17

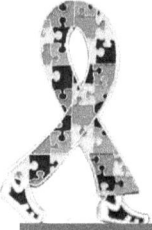

Toilet Training

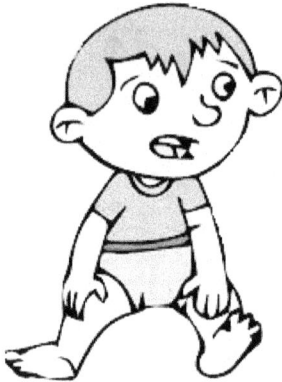

Excretion is a natural life process but that does not mean it is easy and trouble free specially in case of children. Toilet training any child is difficult but toilet training a child in the autism spectrum can particularly be a challenging job. They have various difficulties in accepting the toilet training.

Child anticipating discomfort

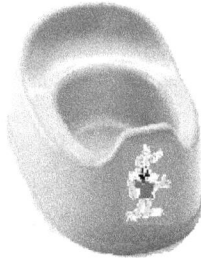

Possible difficulties of a child for accepting toilet training

1. Physical Discomfort

There might be some medical reasons which create physical discomfort during toileting. There might be a difficulty in motor coordination. For example, pulling down the underwear and stepping out of it might be a difficult task for the child.

2. Communication Difficulty

Due to the child's communication problem he/she might not be able to express his urge for toileting.

3. Language Problem

Due to the inability to understand the language the child may not know what is expected from him/her.

4. Sensory Issues

The child might be scared to sit on the toilet seat as he/she might find it too hard/too soft or the noise of the flush might be too loud for him/her.

5. Routine Diversion

Generally children in the autistic spectrum prefer a routine. They do not like anything out of the routine. So changing from diaper to using the toilet is a difficult task for them.

Certain things are to be kept in mind before toilet training a child with ASD.

Points to remember before toilet training the child

1. Begin when your child is ready

The child has to learn the small skills first before giving him toilet training. According to ABA the task of toilet training has to be split into small skills first. Using chaining or prompting, the child has to master the small skills like taking down an underwear, pulling up an underwear, washing hands etc.

2. Ignore the comments of friends, relatives and others

For a typical child toilet training generally starts when the child is around two years old but in a child with ASD it will be too difficult to start at two. So you may hear various negative comments of various people around you. Just ignore them.

3. Inform the full team

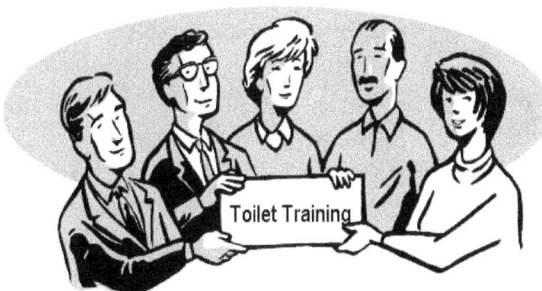

Collaborative effort of team

At the appropriate time (when the child is ready) start the training by informing your full team i.e. parents, grandparents, therapist, teacher as well as any other helper (maid) whom you think should be notified. A child learns better by collaborative effort.

4. Be patient

It's natural to get frustrated at times but always remember *"Each bud takes its time to blossom"*. So your child might learn the skill at a slightly later age. If you loose patience and get irritated it will be more difficult for the child to learn the new skills.

5. Never give up

It might take a couple of months or may be a few years for a child with ASD to be toilet trained but the toileting independence will be a reward which will last lifetime.

6. Be consistent

Regularity and consistency is a must in any kind of teaching. So you have to be consistent even though you do not get the desired result quickly.

Useful tips for toilet training

1. Talk to the pediatrician if there is a medical condition associated with urination or bowel movement. If yes then take the doctor's guidance in overcoming the problem. If there is no medical problem then first try to develop only the motor skills of the child with the help of a therapist.
2. Do not wait for the child to tell you his/her need to go to the toilet. Take him/her to the toilet several times during the day at regular intervals.
3. Make picture cards showing every step of toileting.
4. Try to find out if there are any sensory issues which are troubling the child. For example, if the child finds the toilet light too bright fix a low power bulb.
5. Use the same bathroom and the same words for toileting everyday in order to satisfy the routine behaviour of the child.
6. Use reinforcement for each small correct response. The rewards should be interesting to the child. Even a correct attempt should be rewarded.

7. Make two, day wise toilet chart – one for urination and the other for bowel movement. Mention the date, time, small steps done successfully etc. in the chart. The following format is useful.

Date: _____ Day: _____			
Fluid intake time	**Urination time**	**Taken to the toilet**	**Accidental**

8. Give more fluids like juice, milk, water etc. during toilet training so that the child will have greater need to go to the toilet. The greater the need the more number of times he/she will get the practice. Hence, the probability of getting the desired behaviour will also increase.

9. During visit to the toilet remove the other sensory distractions. For example, switch off the music. Make sure the soap used in the bathroom is not too strong or too mild for the child.

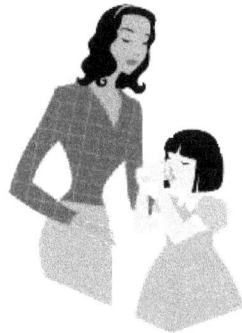

Girl drinking juice

The urination and bowel movement will depend on the fluid intake and the diet of the child. The diet has to be nutritive and well balanced, as per the health and sensory issues of the child.

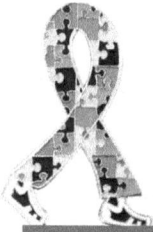

Chapter 18

Nutrition and Diet

According to WHO (World Health Organization) nutrition is the intake of food considered in relation to the body's dietary needs. Good and adequate nutrition, well balanced diet and regular physical activity forms the base of good health. Poor nutrition leads to reduced immunity, increased susceptibility to disease, improper development and reduced productivity.

However, developing healthy food habits in children is an arduous task for most parents. It becomes further difficult if the child has ASD. Just because the child has ASD does not mean that the child will have food sensitivity but if the child gets frequent digestion problem then the parents need to explore the various special diet options.

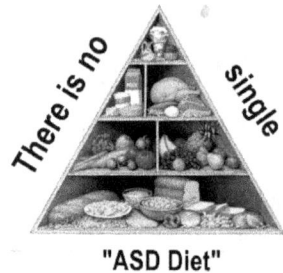

"ASD Diet"

Unfortunately there is no fixed diet for ASD. The different types of diet, needs to be tried on a hit and trial basis. It takes around three to four weeks to know the positive effect of a particular diet.

Types of Diets

The different types of diets which can be tried are:

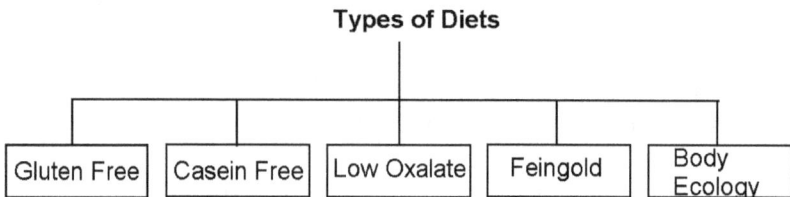

Types of Diets

Gluten Free	Casein Free	Low Oxalate	Feingold	Body Ecology

Various types of diet

Gluten Free

Gluten is the protein present in various grains such as barley, rye, farina (suji), semolina, wheat and wheat products. Gluten causes inflammation in the small intestine of several people and hence causes problems.

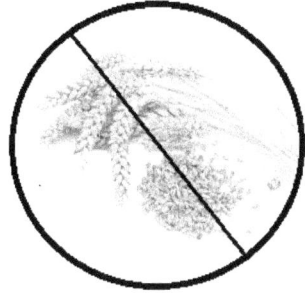

Gluten free diet

Gluten containing food items

Bread, chapati, noodles, biscuit, cake, horlicks, pizza, burger, etc.

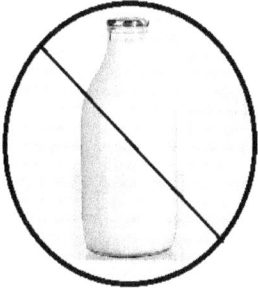

Casein free diet

Casein Free

Casein is the protein present in milk and milk products such as cheese, curd, cottage cheese (paneer) etc.

Casein containing food items

Chocolate, butter, margarine, pudding, many Indian sweets like barfi, rasgulla etc.

Low Oxalate

Oxalates are naturally occurring chemicals present in plants, animals as well as human beings. Oxalates can bind with Calcium and crystallize. This can irritate our body cells and lead to inflammation and pain.

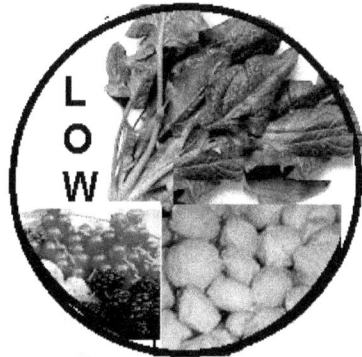

Low oxalate diet

High oxalate food items

Leafy vegetables, soya bean, tofu, grapes, berries, nuts etc.

Feingold

This diet eliminates all food items containing artificial color, artificial flavour, sweetener and preservatives. All such things trigger the hyperactivity in children.

Feingold containing food items

Most ready made food items - chips, biscuits, tinned food, bottled juice, soft drink etc.

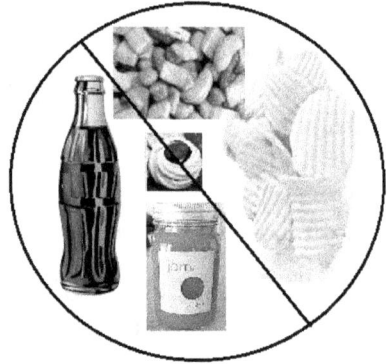

Feingold diet

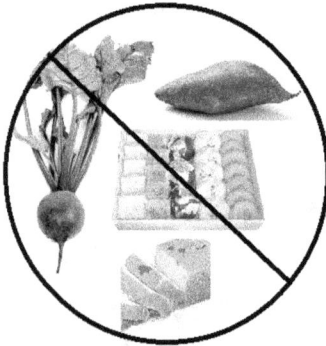

Body ecology diet

Body Ecology

This diet re-establishes the intestinal flora (useful bacteria present in the intestine) and heals the body. It eliminates the yeast and fungal infections of the body which often develops due to the long term intake of several medicines. It eliminates mushroom, refined oil, sweet vegetables and sweets, baked products etc.

Yeast enhancing food items

Honey, molasses (gur), sweets, pea, beetroot, bread, cake, dry fruit etc.

The parents have to do a lot of trial and error to find out the best suited diet for their child.

It is advisable to maintain a day wise diet chart. This would help the parents to determine the comfortable food for their child.

The diet chart can be maintained in the following format:

Daywise Dietchart

Date		Day	
Time	**Food item**	**Symptoms (if any)**	**Degree** **0 = nil** **1 = mild** **2 = moderate** **3 = severe**

The environmental factors can also be added to the chart. By environmental factors I mean the room the child was fed in, the persons who were around, if any music/TV was on etc.

Some general tips

1) Avoid spicy food and junk food.
2) Control fried food.
3) Try one diet at a time.
4) Ensure that the child drinks about 7- 8 glasses of water everyday.

Nutrition supplements

In order to try out the various diets the child may become deficit of certain nutrients. Hence, it is required to use the supplements. It's better to consult a pediatrician before starting any supplement. It would be best if the child can tolerate a multi vitamin but many children have some side effects with multi vitamin.

Supplements with maximum benefit and least side effect

S.No.	Supplement	Benefit
1.	Probiotics(Live useful bacteria)	Helps in improving the intestinal functions. It also improves the immune system
2.	Enzymes	Aids digestion
3.	Magnesium	Healthy nervous system (Overdose may cause diarrhea)
4.	Vitamin D	Strong bones

Note: Consult a pediatrician before starting any supplement.

Apart from the physical sensitivity/allergy the texture of the food might also create problem for children with ASD. For example, they may like crunchy food but may not like mushy food. While trying various diets remember the sensory issues of the child. Along with proper diet, regular exercise and relaxation is also needed by children to reach their full potential.

Chapter 19

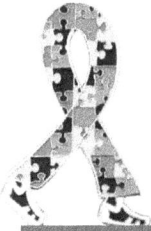

Relaxation and Exercise

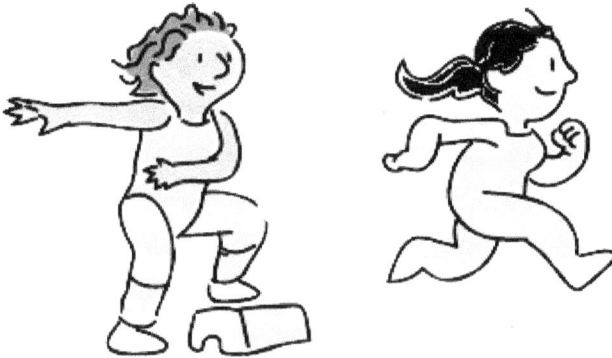

Boy exercising and girl jogging

Exercise is good for every child and every adult in all state of health. It will benefit every child irrespective of his/her position in the autistic spectrum. The physical exercise releases some feel good chemicals known as endorphins in the body which reduces stress, aggression, repetitive behaviour, mouthing, self injury etc. which are common behaviour problems in autism.

Parent's encouragement

The parents need to find out the interest of the child before encouraging them to exercise. The children will be willing to do the exercise only if it is as per their liking. For example, some children may like to run others may like to play in water and gradually learn to swim, still others may like aerobics. Whatever physical activity is enjoyed by the child the parents should preferably join them. This will not only make the parents as role models but children will feel encouraged to continue the activity on a regular basis.

Various relaxation therapies

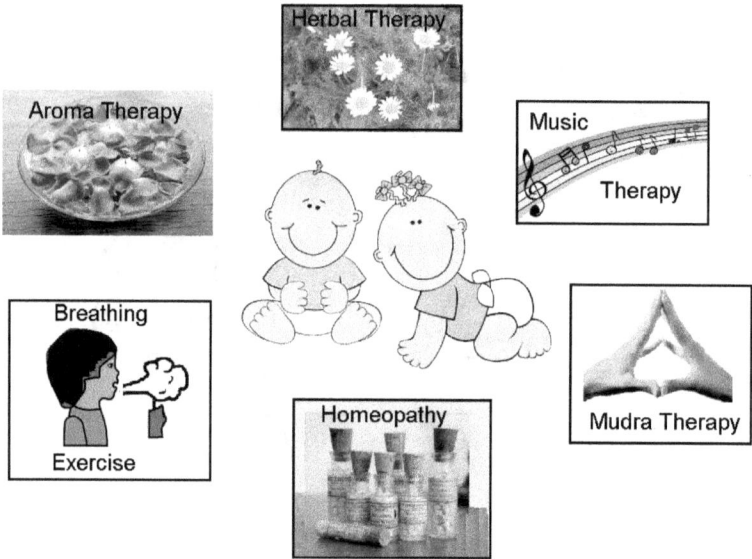

Alternate therapies for relaxation

The various relaxation and healing therapies are mudra therapy, homeopathy, pranayama, aroma therapy, herbal therapy, music therapy, art therapy and animal therapy. The same relaxation method may not work for all the children having similar problems. Even for a particular child different therapies or a combination of therapies may work well at different situations.

a. Mudra Therapy

The human body regularly emits magnetic waves which causes an imbalance in the "Panch bhuta" (five basic elements - air, water, fire, earth and space) present within the body and in the universe. This imbalance causes ailments. Our five fingers in each hand correspond to these five elements. Hence, by using various mudras (postures) of finger tips

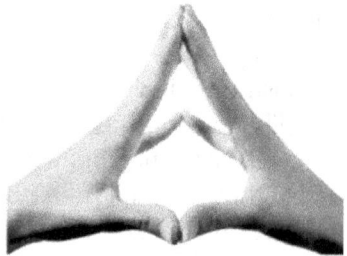

Hakini mudra

and thumb we can restore the balance of the magnetic waves as well as the five basic elements thereby healing our body.

Hakini mudra has a calming effect on the body. To do this mudra, join the tips of four fingers and thumb of one hand with the tips of four fingers and the thumb of the other hand. To get the maximum benefit it should be practiced 15 minutes twice a day (start with less time and gradually increase it).

b. Homeopathy

Homeopathy is a safe and effective healing therapy with rare side effects. Some of the common calming homeopathy medicines are Aconitum Napellus, Calcarea Phosphorica, Natrum Muriaticum and Chamomillia. However, it is advisable to consult a homeopath before trying any medicine.

c. Breathing Exercise (Pranayama)

"Pranayama" is a Sanskrit word which means extension of the life force. It is derived from two words "Prana" meaning life which refers to the breath and "ayama" meaning to extend. Simple breathing exercise can be taught to children using picture cards. Breathe in hold for five seconds; breathe out hold for five seconds.

Benefits of Pranayama

1. It relaxes the muscles.
2. It calms the nerves.
3. It helps to release endorphins the brain chemical which releases stress and reduces pain.

d. Aroma Therapy

The inhalation of essential oils from plants for healing purpose is known as *aromatherapy*. The scientific study at the university of Maryland has proved that aromatherapy with lavender oil relaxes the nerves and soothes the mind. (Incense sticks may be used if essential oils are not available). A light massage with lavender oil also helps many children to calm down.

e. Herbal Therapy

The other name of this therapy is Ayurvedic therapy which uses different parts of plants for healing. The extract from flower of chamomile (Hindi name Babuna) gives a calming effect to the body.

f. Music Therapy

Some of the researchers have found that listening to western classical instrumental music composed by Mozart has a lot of relaxing effect on the children with ASD. This has been termed as *Mozart effect.*

g. Art Therapy

Since proper communication is one of the major problems of autism, art therapy is effective in many individuals. Many children can think and remember in terms of pictures. This therapy can develop motor skills, help to recognize facial expression, help to release stress etc.

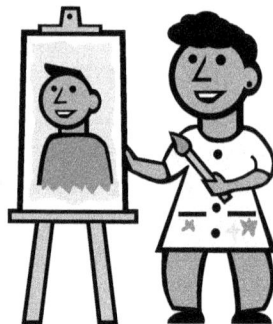
A boy practicing art therapy

h. Animal Therapy

Research shows that domestic animals can relate to these unique children and these children can also relate to animals well although they have a hard time relating to their peer group. So it might be a good idea to keep a pet dog if expenses and other circumstances allow. Pets can be wonderful companions.

I remember Mr. Ramanathan telling me that his son Venu was very attached to their dog. Venu had the habit of wandering. Once the entrance door was not locked properly and Venu went out. The dog followed him. The family panicked when they realized that Venu was missing. They searched him inside the house, around the neighbourhood and all other probable places but could not find him. Venu's mother started crying, Ramanathan informed the police. After three hours the dog sniffed back into the house bringing Venu along with him.

Some of the relaxation therapies like Hakini mudra and Pranayama can be practiced by the entire family together.

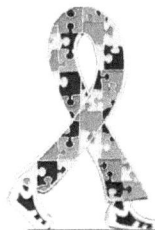

Chapter 20

Sibling and Family

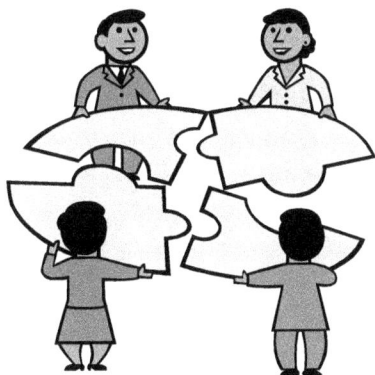

The entire family putting the puzzle pieces together

The diagnosis and confirmation of autism is a life changing event for most parents. The entire family is affected emotionally, physically, financially as well as socially. Our society accepts people with physical disability but is biased against those with neuro developmental disorders. As a result coping becomes difficult most of the time. Families often become socially isolated. Although there is no single rule to come out of it but certain strategies can help.

Some strategies to tackle the special challenges and cherish the joy of parenting

1. Collect as much information as possible for autism.
2. Accept your child. He/She can feel your love. He/She wants to reciprocate it too but does not know how to do it.
3. Appreciate the small victories achieved by your child.
4. There is no right or wrong method of parenting. Do what works for your child.
5. Join some support group.
6. Take a break and spend some quality time with a friend. You need not feel guilty about it.
7. Talk about your feelings with a trusted relative or friend.
8. Be willing to ask for help.
9. Make an educational plan.
10. Make financial plan for the child.

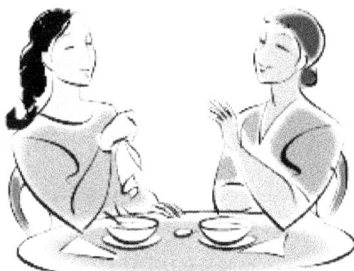

An outing with a friend

11. Pay attention to the other sibling (if any).
12. Don't give up. Focus on what you can control in the moment not what you can't predict or control in future.
13. Do pranayama or some other exercise on a regular basis (even if it is just for ten minutes a day).

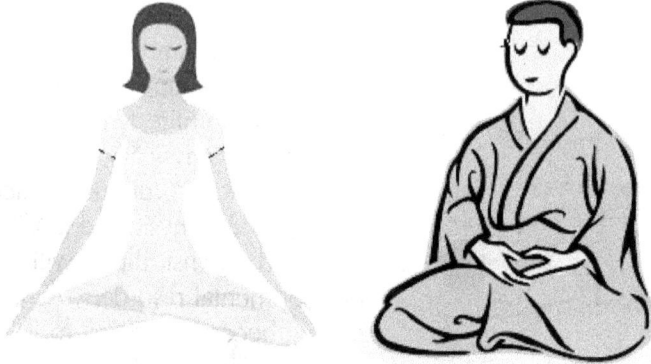

Couple practicing meditation

14. Try to meditate for some time.
15. Remember all your negative feelings are not facts, with your consistent effort the child can progress better than what you can imagine at present.

I remember once I met a mother of a 9 year old autistic boy who told me that her son did not speak a single word till 7 years but she did not give up. Due to her diligence and persistent effort her son spoke the first word "ma" on his eighth birthday. After that he gradually learnt many more words. The doctors were surprised too. I think all of us should have this kind of diligence.

The medicine of love is effective in all kinds of adversities in life. The strong affectionate bond which the parents have with their children whether autistic or typically growing is incomparable.

Raising children is a difficult job for all parents in the modern world. It becomes tougher when one child is typically developing and the other is in the autistic spectrum. Due to the developmental problem the child in the autistic spectrum needs more attention of his/her parents. Even the parents try to put in their best in upbringing their child in the autistic spectrum which is both physically and emotionally exhaustive for them. As a result the typically developing child tends to feel neglected. Let us have a look at their feelings.

Few things the sibling wishes that their parents knew

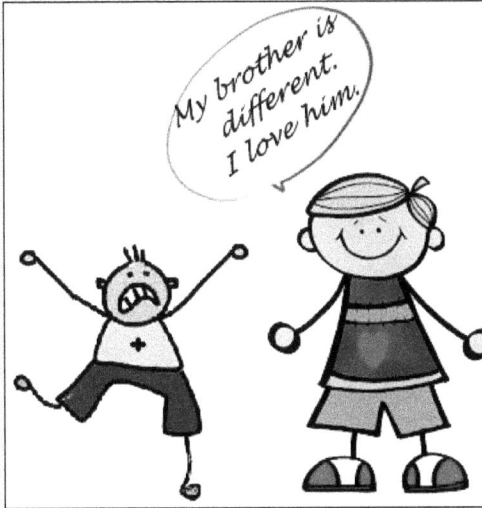

Love of two brothers

1. I need your attention too

Sibling rivalry is common among all children across the world but having a child in the autistic spectrum is a more demanding job for the parents. As a result parents are almost left with very little or no time for the typical child. This results in a feeling of jealousy in the mind of the sibling.

2. I don't understand what's wrong with him/her

Siblings are confused, puzzled and sometimes feel nervous to see the non traditional behaviour of their brother/sister. This might make them vulnerable to psychological problems in their later years of life.

3. I feel embarrassed in front of my friends

Siblings feel awkward in front of their friends since their friends might make fun of the brother/sister due to their lack of knowledge about autism. Siblings are generally protective of their brother/sister. They even feel embarrassed by the unwanted stare of people at public places.

4. I feel sad

The siblings get emotionally affected since they can see that in-spite of a lot of effort their brother/sister is not showing the expected behaviour. They also feel sad when they see the parents react in a different manner for the same behaviour shown by him/her as his/her brother/sister. For example, for showing aggressive behaviour the parents might be tolerant for the autistic child but may loose patience and scold the typically growing child.

5. I feel frustrated

Brothers/sisters are first playmate for any child. As a result the siblings feel frustrated when their autistic brother/sister does not show any interest in playing with them. Even if they show interest they do not understand the rules of the game.

6. I feel tensed

The siblings gradually realize that their parents expect them to make up for the deficit. As a result they feel tensed. Fear and phobia develops in many children.

7. Your stress affects me

The grief and stress of the parents affects the siblings as well. This is sometimes manifested in the form of poor academic performance or lack of appetite or they may start crying for negligible reasons.

Some parenting tips to manage the siblings

1. Set aside some time everyday exclusively for the sibling. Make him/her feel special during that time. During the exclusive time try not to attend any phone calls or text messages. Give him/her the feeling that he/she is equally loved and equally precious to you.
2. Depending upon the age of the sibling try to explain about autism to him/her. You may give the example of a peacock. Tell him/her that even though the peacock is a beautiful bird it cannot fly very high in the sky like the other birds. Similarly even though your brother/sister is a wonderful person he/she is unable to do certain things.
3. Talk to the class teacher/principal of your typically developing child and try to organize an Autism Awareness Day in your child's school. It can be organized on 2nd April since this date is designated as World Autism Awareness Day by the United Nations General Assembly.
4. Explain it to the typical child that he/she is capable of doing much better whereas his/her brother/sister has a limitation.

5. Involve the sibling in creating picture cards or other teaching aids for his brother/sister.
6. Give rewards and praise the good deeds of the typical child along with his brother/sister.
7. It is very natural for the parents to let out their pent up stress onto their typically developing child. It's like the release of the steam in a pressure cooker. Try to share your feelings with your trusted friends. Make a support group of parents of autistic children so that the typical child does not become the victim of your pent up emotions.

One of the problems in a country like India is the overindulgence of relatives. Sometimes they are supportive but many times too many advises from too many relatives becomes stressful. It has to be handled tactfully.

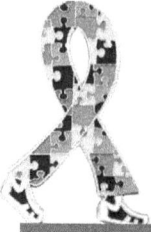

Chapter 21

Friends and Relatives

The diagnosis of autism is often overwhelming for the parents. The dreams and expectations of parenthood are shattered. The lack of communication and social skills leading to a different behaviour with occasional meltdowns leaves parents with a dilemma of whether to socialize with friends/ relatives or not. It becomes difficult for the parents to cope with the stare, unpleasant comments and

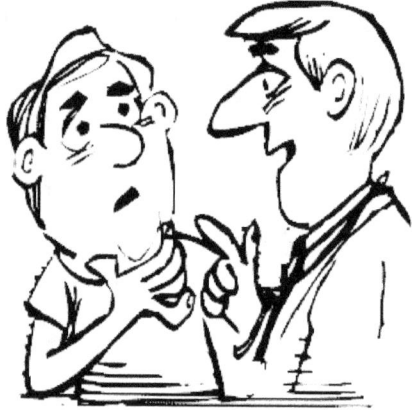

Relative giving advice

questions of friends/relatives. As a result many prefer not to socialize. Social isolation along with the everyday stress of managing the household, raising the autistic child, expensive treatment of the child, lack of sleep etc. leads to frustration, anxiety and depression of the parent.

In my opinion parents should try to educate their friends and relatives. Those who care for you would love to know more about autism and share your feelings; those who don't want to know do not deserve your lovely company.

Even while going for a walk or going to the market the child can be taken along. Those who stare on the way can be handed over an awareness card like the following:

PUBLIC AUTISM AWARENESS CARD

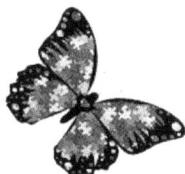

I am sorry if my child's behaviour is bothering you. It is not his/her lack of discipline.

He/She has autistic spectrum disorder (ASD).

Autism is a lifelong developmental disorder which is NOT contagious.

1 in 68 children have ASD. **My child is that one.**

The three main areas of difficulty of children with autism are -
communication, socialization and behaviour skills.

Accept
Understand
Love

My child is trying to cope, please don't stare or be judgemental.

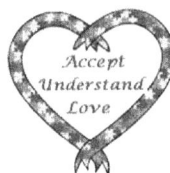

Awareness card

Many times the caring friends and relatives want to help but do not know how to do so.

Some suggestions for the caring friends and relatives

1. Read this book.
2. Make autism awareness cards and spread the awareness.
3. Be a patient listener.
4. Give moral encouragement.
5. Volunteer to do some chore for your friend/relative. For example, when you go to buy your own grocery you can buy it for your friend/relative as well.
6. Make picture cards for the child to develop his/her everyday skills.

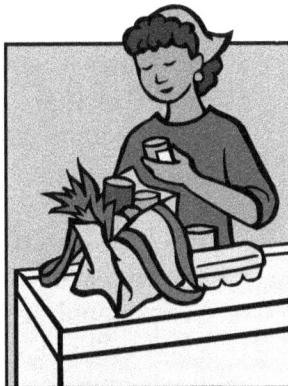

A friend helping with grocery

7. Give extra attention to the typical sibling (They often feel neglected).
8. Gather information about the support group in your friend's/relative's locality.
9. Appreciate the achievements of the child. For example, if a child can look at the picture of glass of water and point at it or pick up the glass even at the age of six it is a big achievement for him/her.
10. Accompany your friend/relative to the doctor's visit whenever possible.

10 Things Every Parent with their child in the autistic spectrum would like to hear

1. **What people commonly say:** "Do you know whose family the autism came from?"
   Fact: The exact cause of autism is still under research. There is no single cause. Gene mutation could be just one of the causes.
   It's better to say: "I am here if you want to talk.'

2. **What people commonly say:** "What is the future of your child?"
   Fact: Every child in the autistic spectrum is unique. It is not possible to predict the future.
   It's better to say: "I am always there with you."

3. **What people commonly say:** "You must not be getting any time for yourself."
   Fact: Since every child behaves in a unique manner it is very challenging and exhaustive for the parents.
   It's better to say: "Can you find out some time when we can sit and chat or go out for a little while?"

4. **What people commonly say:** "Life does not give us anything we cannot handle."
   Fact: Having a child lying in the autistic spectrum is neither the choice nor the fault of the parents.
   It's better to say: "Can I do anything for you?"

5. **What people commonly say:** "You should have taken your child to the doctor earlier. May be then he/she would have been cured."
   Fact: The warning signs can develop at any age up to five

years. The cure for autism is yet to be discovered.

It's better to say: "What all can I do to make his/her life more comfortable?"

6. **What people commonly say:** "I don't know how you do it, had I been at your place I couldn't/wouldn't have done it."

Fact: You cannot judge someone until you get into their shoes.

It's better to say: "Please tell me how can I interact with your child."

7. **What people commonly say:** "You pamper your child too much. You need to be strict with him/her and teach him/her some discipline."

Fact: Children lying in the autistic spectrum have difficulty in communication skills and as a result have difficulty in understanding things.

It's better to say: "Is there any method by which communication becomes easy for your child?'

8. **What people commonly say:** "Your child does not look like he/she has autism."

Fact: There is no particular look for autism. It is often referred as invisible disability. The child may not have any distinguishable physical impairment but may have some physical problems associated with autism.

It's better to say: "Your child looks adorable."

9. **What people commonly say:** "Why don't you take your child for ayurvedic /homeopathic treatment? I know of a person who got cured."

Fact: There is no definite treatment. Every child reacts differently to the medicines.

It's better to say: "I read/heard about an alternative effective treatment, if you would like I can share it with you."

10. **What people commonly say:** "What special talent does your child have?"

Fact: Every child is not a savant.

It's better to say: "How is your child doing?"

Many friends and relatives want to interact with the autistic child but feel uncomfortable in doing so since they are unsure of what to say or do. Here are some ideas.

10 Ways to connect with an autistic child

1. Get to know the likes and dislikes of the child through the parent.
2. Respect the parent's wishes and the needs of the child.
3. Be aware of the child's sensory issues.
4. Use short simple words.
5. Try to go down at the mental level of the child irrespective of his/her age.
6. Try to build a routine. For example, every time you meet the child just say hello. Don't change it to Hi or How are you etc.
7. Try to help them not control them.
8. Do not expect eye contact from the child.
9. Do not assume that the child lacks emotions.
10. Do not compare with others.

Children with autism thrive on set schedules. Going for a vacation in a new place away from home disrupts their routine hence, it causes discomfort. This can be overcome by proper planning and organizing.

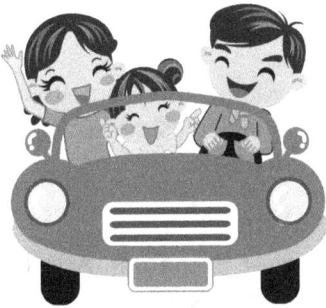
Family going on a vacation

Vacation Planning

The key to any enjoyable vacation is planning ahead. All of us have to adjust to certain things during vacation like change of environment, change of routine, delay at the airport/railway station or on the road etc. These changes often become very stressful for the families having a member in the autistic spectrum. For many parents it turns out to be a combination of disappointment and frustration.

Even if the vacation is at the child's grandparent's house certain preparations will make the adjustments easier for the autistic child.

10 Strategies for an enjoyable vacation

1. Prepare your child

Two to three weeks prior to the trip start showing pictures, brochures, videos of the destination place to the child so that the child becomes familiar with the place.

2. Make arrangements ahead of time

Inform the hotel and the airlines/railways about your child's condition ahead of time. You can give them an awareness booklet.

3. Select the mode of transportation carefully

Depending on the comfort factor of the child the mode of transportation needs to be selected. For example, the train journey is cheaper but it takes a long time. The child may not feel comfortable for long. On the other hand the plane journey is expensive but takes a short time. I would suggest the first journey whether by plane or train should be for a short distance. The problems faced in this can be overcome in the next trip.

4. Prepare the identification and awareness cards

A number of identity cards and awareness cards needs to be prepared before the trip. Ensure that an identity card is always pinned up in the child's clothes. It can also be attached to a sling and put around the neck.

5. Pack the essential items

If the child is on a special diet carry it with you for the journey and notify the hotel in advance. Pack your child's medicines, sensory toys if any, favourite picture books, favourite toiletries etc.

6. Medical check up before the vacation

Arrange for a medical check up few days prior to the trip. Ask the doctor to prescribe some medicine for travel sickness and some medicine to keep the child calm during the journey.

7. Medical file and letter from the child's physician

A letter from the child's physician mentioning his/her health condition and needs will help in getting proper seat in the train or plane. In case, you are travelling by plane this letter will make the security check easier. Carrying the child's medical file will come in use just in case there is some emergency and there is a need to consult the local doctor.

8. Take care of sensory issues of the child

As per the requirement of the child use sunglasses, earplug or headphone, chewing gum, stress balls etc. during the journey.

9. Ease transition

As far as possible make the furniture arrangement of the hotel room according to your house. For example, if the bed is touching the wall in your child's room request the hotel staff to shift the bed. Carry the comfortable pillow and blanket of the child. Make sure the power of the bulb is almost the same as your house. This will make the child feel comfortable.

10. Stick to sleep time as far as possible

After the journey try to make the child sleep. Everyday during the vacation try to make the child sleep at his/her normal sleep hours. Adjustment to the new environment will be easier for the child if he/she gets proper rest.

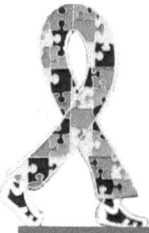

Chapter 23

Adulthood and Career

The transition from adolescent to adulthood can create excitement as well as nervousness in individuals with autism. A parental support as well as advance preparation can make them comfortable. As an advance preparation, parents can encourage their children to try out tasks which are out of their comfort zone. With support they can continue to learn and develop throughout their lives.

As with typical young adults even those in the autistic spectrum need guidance about their further education and job selection.

Some adults with ASD feel comfortable taking up a full time job working with typical adults while others prefer a part time job. Still others prefer to work from home.

Amazing Fact

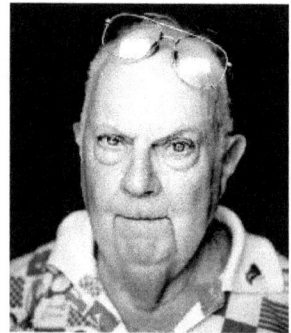

Donald Gary Triplett (born September 1933), the first child diagnosed with autism by Leo Kanner faced many challenges throughout his life but with his family support and his own perseverance he finished his bachelor's degree and later worked in a bank.

Vivekananda has said – *"Purity, patience and perseverance are the three essentials to success and above all love."*

Donald Gary Triplett the first child diagnosed with autism

The decision of further study after schooling will depend upon the interest, ability, sensory need as well as availability of the course. Some adults can excel at vocational studies which include creativity like ceramic work, paper work, stitching work, cooking etc. while others do better at studies involving numbers like statistics, accounts, mathematics etc. Still others may be good at photography, cartoon drawing, graphic designing etc.

Some of the problems faced by autistic adults in the job market are:

- ✗ They might have inadequate language development.
- ✗ Sensory overload might be a problem for them.
- ✗ They generally don't feel comfortable in a crowd.
- ✗ Social interaction might be uncomfortable.

Teaching job is not suitable

Any job that requires inter personal skill is not suitable for individuals with autism.

Some of the jobs not suitable for autistic adults are:

Teaching
School teacher, Lecturer, Professor

Hospitality
Waiter, cashier, receptionist and all other hotel jobs, all kinds of travel and tourism jobs, Front office jobs

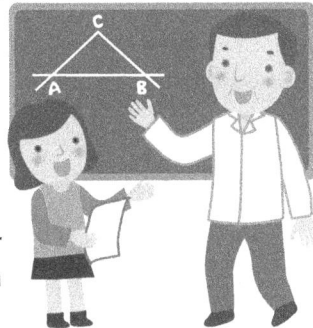

Sales and Marketing
Salesman, sales manager, shopkeeper, ticketing, insurance agents

Beauty
Beautician, barber, make up man

Some employers view autism as an asset and not as a deficiency.

Some of the traits which are beneficial in the job market are

- ✗ Intense focus
- ✗ High level of concentration
- ✗ Need for being systematic
- ✗ Need for following routine
- ✗ Attention to details
- ✗ View from a different perspective

Some of the suitable fields are:

Information Technology-
Computer programmer, Data entry operator, Web designer, Software tester, Software debugger

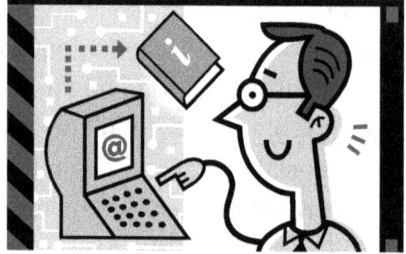

Information technology is a suitable job field

Science
Scientist, Statistician, Mathematician, Veterinarian's assistant, Pathological laboratory assistant, Science or Mathematics editor in publishing industry

Industry
Manufacturing and Packaging, Inventory controller

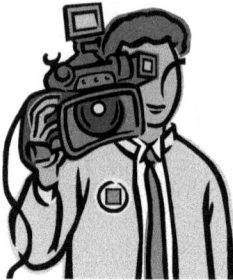

Photographer is a suitable job

Creative
Graphic Designer, Photographer, Animation artist, Commercial artist, Digital designer, Textile designer

Banking and Commerce
Accountant, Bookkeeping, Bank clerk/officer

Assistants
Library assistant, Research assistant, Pharmacy assistant

Music
Instrumentalist, musician

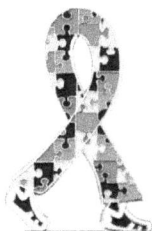

Chapter 24

Dos and Don'ts in ASD

Dos

1. Be kind and compassionate.
2. Be patient while talking to an autistic individual. Talk slowly.
3. Use simple language and small sentences.
4. Teach and encourage individual sports and not team sports. For example, encourage bowling, badminton etc. and not cricket, football.
5. Give little reminders for different activities. For example, remind them to wash hands before eating.
6. Restrict TV viewing time.
7. Avoid soft drinks and junk food.
8. Help your child cope.
9. Designate a calm down space in the house.
10. Explain everything in advance. Let him/her know the schedule in advance especially if there is going to be any change.
11. Try to mimic an outing at home.
12. Prepare a child before a doctor visit.
13. Minimize waiting time at the doctor's clinic with prior appointment. Carry your child's sensory stimulating toy.
14. Explain that the doctor will touch him/her during the visit. Use pictures, diagrams, story books with pictures or a toy doctor set.

Doctor examining a patient

15. Be aware that the adolescence is not affected by autism. All the physical changes take place same as the typical children.
16. Give a positive feedback. Say praise words when the child does a good job even though small. Decide on giving small rewards.

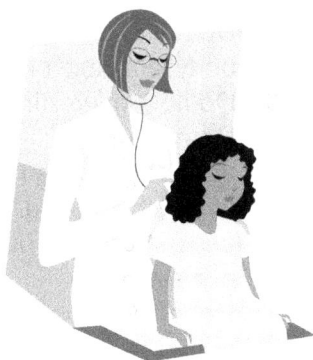

17. Provide visual support.
18. Be ready to help in unexpected ways.
19. Give unconditional love.
20. Try to understand the behaviour of autistic children. Behaviour is always communicative.
21. Always be supportive never judgemental.
22. Believe in your own strength to raise your unique child.
23. Maintain a daily diary of the child.
24. Encourage the special interest of the child.
25. Take care of the sensory issues of your child.

Don'ts

"What seems impossible today, may not be tomorrow."

– Thomas Edison

1. Do not believe nothing can be done.
2. Don't compare one child with the other. Every child is unique.
3. Don't ignore individuals with autism just because they are different.
4. Don't ignore the strengths of autistic children.
5. It is better not to use multiple languages with autistic children. It creates more confusion.
6. Do not make any assumption about the child.
7. Do not expect the child to adjust with his sensory issues.
8. Do not expect the child to understand your facial expression, body language or your tone of voice.
9. Do not underestimate the ability of the child.
10. Do not assume if the child is not able to talk clearly he cannot hear or does not understand what is being said. The child may understand fully but may not be expressive.
11. Do not give surprises. Adaptation to change is very difficult for persons with autism.
12. Do not expect the child to eat the same food if the presentation is changed. He/she may have sensory issues with the food. For

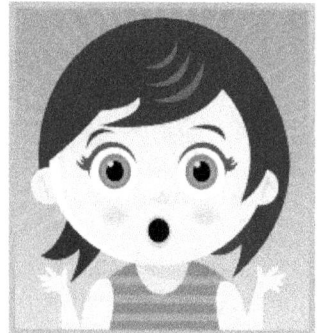

A girl distressed by a surprise

example, the texture or smell might be troublesome for him/her.

13. Do not exempt the child from the rule of sharing and caring.

14. Do not get annoyed by strange reactions or comments.

15. Do not tease or criticize autistic children.

16. Do not give many choices, that creates confusion in autistic individuals.

17. Do not react negatively even if the child does not response to your emotion.

18. Do not force children to socialize.

19. Do not yell or scream. Loud voices may increase their anxiety.

20. Don't try any new medicine just because it claims high or has good advertisement. Take an expert opinion first.

21. Don't consider your child to be a liability. With early intervention and your guidance he/she can be an asset.

22. Don't panic.

23. Don't give up.

24. Don't lose hope.

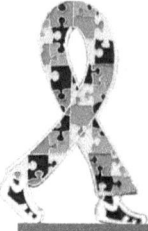

Chapter 25

Frequently Asked Questions

1. **What are the chances of having a second child with autism if my first child is autistic?**
    According to Centre for Disease Control (CDC), parents who have a child with ASD have 2% - 18% chance of having a second child affected. However, since one of the factors of autism is genes and genetic counselling is not available in India no doctor will be able to give guarantee to families about the second child not being affected.

2. **Can autism be screened with prenatal testing?**
    At present there is no test to detect autism in the foetus.

3. **Is brain MRI and EEG always necessary to diagnose and treat autism?**
    No. Autism is diagnosed with the help of developmental screening test and Diagnostic and Statistical Manual of Mental Disorders *(DSM-5, Refer chapter 4)*. However, if there are clinical reasons like seizures or head injury or repeated spells of unconsciousness then MRI and EEG is suggested by the neurologist.

4. **I have never done harm to anyone. Why am I being punished with an autistic child?**
    First of all raising an autistic child is not "worse" than raising a typical child. The perspective of upbringing has to be different. Secondly, there are many couples who go to various doctors, religious places, spiritual leaders etc. in order to have a child but remain unsuccessful. You are lucky to have a loving child. Enjoy your parenthood. Finally, your child is not a punishment but a blessing. He/she is more spiritual oriented, hence tries to cut off the communication and socialization distractions. There are many things which you can learn from your child.

5. **What is the difference between girls and boys with autism?**
    Boys are more likely to have autism than girls (5:1 ratio)

but girls with autism have greater learning disabilities and academic problems as compared to the boys. The girls have less sensory irritability and also engage in fewer repetitive behaviours.

6. **My daughter is 8 years old. She is very shy and talks less right from her childhood. She bends her head while talking to show respect. Is it possible for her to develop autism at this age?**

   Extreme shyness masked the ASD symptom of lack of social interaction. Bending head could be the inability to make eye contact which is one of the common symptoms of autism. Hence the doctor probably missed the early diagnosis. Moreover the specific interest in girls is generally with dolls, princesses or drawing which is common in typically growing children. So it is quite possible for the pediatrician to miss out ASD.

7. **Should I tell my child that he/she has autism?**

   Yes. Autism is neither a disease nor a degenerative illness. It is a disorder (set of symptoms) which makes an individual different. I think you will agree with me that it would be worse if a child hears from someone else that he/she has autism when he/she does not even know what it means. So it's better that the parents explain the situation to their children.

8. **What is the right age to tell children that they have autism?**

   There is no right age. It will depend on the child's developmental level, his/her environment and personal family circumstances.

9. **How should I explain autism to my child?**

   It cannot be explained in a single day. The explanation has to be a continuous process. Plant the seeds by explaining the diversity that exists among people like different types of hair, complexion, height etc. Explain the similarities as well like we all eat food, take bath etc. Gradually highlight the positive qualities of your child to him/her and explain that he/she thinks differently. He/she is unique and special which in other words is known as autism.

10. **What is the difference between mental retardation and autism?**

Individuals with mental retardation (now known as intellectual impairment) have below average intellectual capability while individuals with autism have average to above average intelligence quotient (IQ). However, since communication is a problem area of ASD and communication skills are an integral part of most intelligence tests many times autistic individuals are misdiagnosed with mental retardation.

11. **My son is 9 years old, with early intervention programme my son is now able to read alphabets and numbers but why is he not able to write them?**

Research shows that children with autism can space, size and align their letters and numbers. However, they have a great difficulty in forming the letters and numbers due to their lack of fine motor skills.

12. **How can I develop the fine motor skills of my child?**

Make him play with plastercine, squeeze out water from a sponge, put a string inside colourful beads (big ones), do some finger painting and paper folding projects.

13. **My daughter is 12 years old. She has improved a lot with early intervention. Should I admit her to the regular school now?**

I won't recommend you to do that since she is in her adolescent year. As such she will have to face a lot of new challenges. Sending her to a regular school at this stage might become too much for her to handle. It might lead to regression.

14. **Is there any institution in India which organizes parent's training programme for autism?**

Yes.

i. Behaviour Momentum India. They have branches in Bangalore, Delhi, Kolkata, Lucknow and Mumbai.
Web:http://behaviormomentum.com/services/parent-training/

ii. Action for Autism- They organize many workshops, trainings as well as diploma courses.

Web: http://www.autism-india.org/customized-trainings

15. I am getting a transfer from my office. Are there any precautions which we need to take for our son?

As far as possible try to create a similar environment. This will make adjustments easier for your son. For example, if you live on the first floor, rent/buy a first floor house in the new location. Start preparing your son in advance. Get pictures of the new house, surroundings etc. in advance and show them to your son.

16. A friend told me that all children with autism get seizure at some stage of life. Is it true?

No. All children with autism do not get seizure disorder. Only around 20-25% of children with autism develop seizures which can be controlled with proper medicines.

17. Can autistic adults get married?

This will depend on the ability and personal choice of the individual. Many high functional autistic adults are married and leading a happy life.

18. Will my son be able to drive when he is 21?

This will depend on your child's coordination of motor skills, ability to focus and understanding of the other vehicles on the road.

19. My husband and I want to go out once in a while without our son. Is it okay to do so?

If you have someone trustworthy who can take care of your child's special needs then you need not feel guilty in going out. You can take care of your son only when you take care of yourself properly.

20. Who will take care of our child when we are not there?

This is the most frightening question for all parents. The first thing you need to plan is for the financial security of the child. Talk to a lawyer and make a will. Appoint some legal guardian (any trusted friend or relative) for your child. Train that person and let him/her interact with your child right from now.

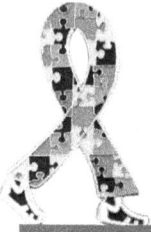

Chapter 26

Resource List

No doubt the diagnosis of autism is overwhelming for the parents but it is a diagnosis not a dead end. Although hopelessness, anger, frustration etc. are common emotions but these emotions won't change the situation. So it would be more practical to do the best in the given situation. One of the most important things is to make the financial plan since the various treatment methods are quiet expensive. One

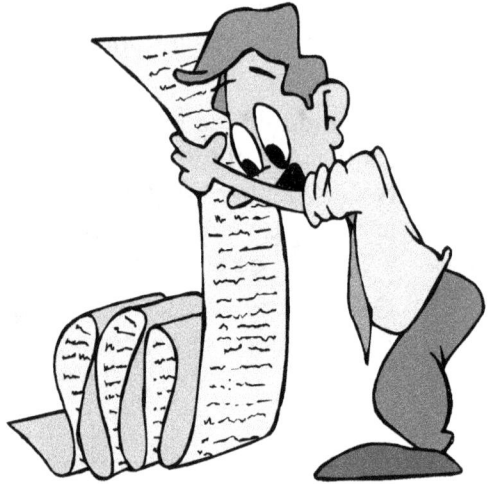

A man looking into the resource list

of the best insurance scheme is "Niramaya Scheme".

Niramaya Scheme

Nirmaya Scheme is an affordable Health Insurance Scheme for the welfare of persons with Autism, Cerebral Palsy, Mental Retardation and Multiple Disabilities.

Special Features of Niramaya Scheme

1. It is open for all. There is no restriction of income, age, caste, or religion.
2. There is a single premium across age band.
3. There is no pre medical check up.
4. There is no exclusion of the pre existing conditions.

5. The insurance coverage is up to Rs. One lakh/annum.
6. The scheme is available all over India except Jammu and Kashmir.
7. The service ranges from regular medical check up to hospitalization.

Niramaya Coverage Chart

Overall Limit for Hospitalization	**1,00,000/-**
Hospitalization	1,00,000/-
Corrective surgery	50,000/-
Non Surgical	15,000/-
Preventive surgery	15,000/-
Overall Limit for Out Patient Dept.	**10,000/-**
OPD treatment including tests	5,000/-
Regular medical checkup	5,000/-
On-going Therapies	10,000/-
Dental Preventive Dentistry	2,500/-
Alternative Medicine (IPD and OPD)	4,500/-
Transportation Costs (IPD and OPD)	1,000/-
ANNUAL INSURANCE COVER	**1,00,000/-**

Enrolment

Any eligible person can apply for enrolment under the scheme through the nearest organization registered with the National Trust. (Check the registered organizations at the website under Regd. NGO's heading).

Address of the Head Office

National Trust

Ministry of Social Justice and Empowerment
16B, Bada Bazar Road, Old Rajinder Nagar
New Delhi 110060
Tel: 011–43187878, 43187878

There are branches in different states.
For details check the website:
www.niramayascheme.com

Autism Specific Schools and Organizations in India (listed by Union Territory)

Andaman and Nicobar

Disha
Rangat
Beside Methodist Church
School Middle Andaman
District – Andaman 744205
Tel: 03192 275184

Chandigarh

Advance Rehabilitation Center
House Number 7
Sector 15A, Chandigarh

Tel: 95011 22777, 90414 00677
Email: therapychd@gmail.com
Web: www.therapychd.com

New Delhi and NCR

Action For Autism (AFA)
The National Centre for Autism

Pocket 7 & 8 Jasola Vihar
New Delhi-110025
Tel: 011– 65347422, 40540991, 40540992
Email: actionforautism@gmail.com

Vatsalya Special School
R-756 Old Rajinder Nagar
New Delhi
Tel: 011– 25862824

SOCH
7517 (Basement), DLF Phase 4,
Near Supermart 2, Gurgaon
Tel: 9910199877,
981088 7523, 9818112646,
9540247551
Email: msamnani77@gmail.com
Web: www.sochindia.org

St. Mary's School, Aasmaan
Sector-19, Dwarka
New Delhi 110 075
Tel: 011– 28042487
Email: st.marys.19@gmail.com
Web: www.
stmarysschooldwarka.in/
inclusive_education/aasmaan

Ashish Centre
Plot number 26B Sulahkul Vihar
(behind Sulahkul Mandir)
Old Palam-Kakrola Road,
Near 14B sector Dwarka,
New Delhi-110078
Tel: 011– 65029394, 65029395
Email: mail@ashishindia.org
Web: www.ashishindia.org

Rajkumari Amrit Kaur Child
Study Centre Department of
Child Development
Lady Irwin College
Sikandra Road, New Delhi
Tel: 011– 23719859, 23318850
Email: rakcsc.lic@gmail.com
Web: http://www.ladyirwin.edu.in

Autism Center - School of Hope
(Tamana Association)
CPWD Complex Near Chinmaya
Vidyalaya Vasant Vihar
New Delhi 110 057
Tel: 011 – 26143843, 26153474
Email: schoolofhope@
tamana.org
Web: http://www.tamana.org/
AutismCenter.aspx

Orkids Punjabi Bagh
14A/53B Punjabi Bagh
(West) New Delhi
Tel: 011– 3222 4456
Web: www.orkidsped.com

**Autism Specific Schools and
Organisations in India** (listed by
State)

Andhra Pradesh
Aarambh
#8-3-966/27, Behind Ameerpet-
Kamma Sangham
Nagarjuna Nagar

Yellareddy Guda Hyderabad,
Andhra Pradesh - 500 073
Tel: 96180 76870, 99667 82332
Email: aarambhyd@gmail.com
Web: http://www.aarambh-

autism.org

Autism Society of Andhra
Pradesh (ASAP)
Ananya Centre for Special
Children Pravara Educational
Trust
1-2-593/26/A, Lane 4, Street 4
Gagan Mahal, Hyderabad,
Andhra Pradesh - 500029
Tel: 040 – 64502596,
98485 13192
Email: autismsociety.
hyderabad@gmail.com
Web: www.asap.org.in

Institute for Remedial
Intervention Services (IRIS)
8-2-/B/2/D Road No:11
Banjara Hills Hyderabad,
Andhra Pradesh - 500034
Tel: 044- 2233-1421
Email: mythilyautism@gmail.com
Web: http://www.autismindia.
com

Parents Association for Autistic
Children (PAAC)
Plot No 115 Defence Colony
Sainikpuri Secunderabad,
Andhra Pradesh -500094
Tel: 040 – 27110749,
94402 49399, 92471 65760
Email: paac2004autism@yahoo.
com, autismpaac@yahoo.co.in
Web: http://paacindia.org

Asperger India
36-136-28, Plot No. 751
G-2, Varun Vihar,
Defence Colony Secunderabad,

Andhra Pradesh 500594
Tel: 040 – 27113317
Email: drmsreenivas@
aspergerindia.com
Web: http://www.aspergerindia.
com

Autism Friendly School
128 Asha Officers Colony
R.K Puram,
Secunderabad 500056
Tel: 040 – 6451 2310,
90320 02310
Email: autisticsociety@gmail.com
www.autisticsocietyofindia.org

Development Centre for
Children with Autism
1143 Siddartha Campus (Beside
Axis Bank) Srinagar Colony
Hyderabad – 500073
Tel: 040–23732285
Email: dccautism@gmail.com
Web: dccautism.org

Supportive Learning Centre
(SLC)
Plot No. 21A, Aurobindo
Colony, Lane 2 Opposite
Reddy Labs J.P Nagar Miyapur
Hyderabad – 500049
Tel: 96185 62396
Email: slcentre2012@gmail.com
Web: autismslc.com

Assam

Assam Autism Foundation
10 Anandam, Lokeshwar
Baruah Path Near FCI gate
New Guwahati, Noonmati,
Assam – 781020

Tel: 97060 14608
Email: autisassam@gmail.com,
shabinaloveschildren@gmail.
com
Web: http://www.aaf.org.in

Bihar

2H/77 Bahadurpur Housing
Colony Near TV Tower,
Bhootnath Road Patna,
Bihar – 800 026
Tel: 98016 99547
Email: utkarshsevasansthan@
gmail.com
*Web:*www.utkarshsevasanthan.in

J.M Institute of Speech and
Hearing
Road No. – 5 Indrapuri
P.O – Keshari Nagar
Patna, Bihar 800 024
Tel: 612 2264805, 612 6414441
Email: info@jminstitute.com
Web: jminstitute.com

Chattisgarh

Sarthak Training Centre for
the Mentally Handicapped
Adarsh Bal Mandir Campus,
Behind Amar Talkies, Dhamtari,
Chattisgarh – 493 773
Asha Ki Kiran School for
the Mentally Handicapped
Teachers' Colony,
Karora Road Tilda, Raipur
Chattisgarh – 493 114

Manovikas Special School
Aghanpur, Dharampura,
Bastar, Chattisgarh – 494 005

Goa

Diuli Daycare Centre cum
Preschool
841/1, Alto Porvorim,
Goa - 403 521
Tel: 0832 - 2414916

Jyot School for Children with
Autism C/o Jimmy Mathai
Opposite Corporation Bank
Behind Nilkunj Heights
Vidyanagar Margao,
Goa - 403601
Tel: 0832 - 2765097
Email: jyotgoa@gmail.com

Gujarat

Disha (Special School and
Autism Centre)
62, Sampat Rao Colony,
Alkapuri Vadodara
Gujarat- 390 007
Tel: 0265 - 2325250, 2356648
Email: dishaautismcentre@
yahoo.com, dishatrustbaroda@
gmail.com
Web: http://www.disha.org/

Haryana

Orkids Panchkula
House No. 14, 2nd Floor
Sector 15 Panchkula Haryana
Tel: 0172 - 3246445
Web: orkidsped.com

Orkids Gurgaon
A 873 A Sushantlok 1 Gurgaon
Tel: 0124 - 6490996
Web: orkidsped.com

Himachal Pradesh

Udaan
C - 35, Sector 2 Bus Stand
New Shimla 171 009
Tel: 177 - 267 2216
Email: udaanhp@gmail.com
Web: udaanshimla.org

Jharkhand

Deepshikha Institute for Child
Development and Mental
Health Arya Samaj Mandir
Swami Shradhanand Road
Ranchi 834 001
Tel: 0651 - 2214203, 2207161
Email: deepshikhainfo@gmail.
com
Website: www.deepshikhaindia.
org

Karnataka

Autism Society of India
60 Vittal Mallya Road
Bangalore 560001
*Tel:*080-41511345,9845953473
Email: autismsociety@gmail.com
Website:
www.autismsocietyofindia.org

Academy for Severe Handicaps
and Autism (ASHA)
L-76/A, Kirloskar Colony,
HBCS 3rd Stage, 4th Block,
Basaveswaranagar,
Bangalore - 560 079
Tel: 080 - 23225279, 23230357
Email: info@ashaforautism.com
Web: http://www.ashaforautism.
com

Akshadhaa Foundation
235, 3rd Main, 4th Block
HBR Layout Bangalore – 560043
Email:
info@akshadhaafoundation.org
Web:
www.akshadhaafoundation.org

Bubbles Centre for Autism
No. 102, Bidarahalli Hobli
Billeshi valle Village
(Beside Shaneeshwara Temple,
Billishivale)
Bangalore – 560077
Tel: 080 –28465336,
94490 03602, 98455 57115
Email: admin@bubblesblr.org
Web: www.bubblesautism.in

Communication DEALL
224,6th A Main, II Block
HRBR Layout Bangalore 560043
Tel: 080 – 2580 0826,
2580 0827, 94803 34809
Email: communicationdeall@
gmail.com
Web: http://www.
communicationdeall.org

Diagnostic and Rehabilitation
Service C/o Spastics Society of
Karnataka
31, 5th Cross, Off 5th Main
Indira Nagar Bangalore 560038
Tel: 080 – 4074 5900

SAI-Apoorva Center for Autism
c/o Lions Club of Sarakki
21st Main, 1st Cross, Marenhalli
JP Nagar Phase 2

Bangalore – 560078
Tel: 94483 72002, 87627 80445
Email:
apoorva@SAIautismcenter.org
Web:
http://www.saiautismcenter.org

Sunshine Autism Trust
280, 6th Cross
Domlur Layout
Bangalore – 560 071
Tel: 080 – 65360892
Email: sunshineautism@gmail.
com
Web: http://www.
autismbangalore.org

Madhya Pradesh

Arushi No.1, Shivaji Nagar
Near MPEB Office
Bhopal – 462016
Tel: 755 4293399, 755 2550827
Email: arushiorg@gmail.com
Web: arushi-india.org

Kerala

Autism Society Thrissur
Sopanam, Greenway,
Chelakottukara
Thrissur East P.O Thrissur District
Kerala - 18
Tel: 9447991406, 94476
68693, 94479 94142
Email: info@
autismsocietythrissur.com
Web: www.
autismsocietythrissur.com

Maharashtra

Forum For Autism
Ground floor, Sorabha house
(Off Colaba causeway)
Mumbai 400 005
Tel: 022–3294 9595
Email: forumforautism@gmail.com
Web: http://forumforautism.org

Ummeed Child Development
Center
1-B, 1/62, Mantri Pride Building
Subhash Nagar, N.M. Joshi Marg
Lower Parel(E) near Arthur Road
Junction Mumbai 400011
Tel: 022 – 65528310,
65564054, 23002006
Email: info@ummeed.org
Web: http://www.ummeed.org

SOPAN
A-4 Silver Arch Haridas Nagar
Borivali (W)
Mumbai 400 092
Tel: 98929 77416, 93232 02768
Email: info@sopan.org,
samarpan@sopan.org
Web: http://www.sopan.org

AARAMBH (Centre for Autism
& Slow Learners)
No.24, Mhada Colony, Near
Shahanurmiya Darga,
Aurangabad
Tel: 82752 84178, 91453 81228
Email: ambikanidhu@gmail.com
Web: aarambhtrust.com

Manbol Autism Center
Ashirwad Bungalow

N-3 , Cidco Near to Ganpati
Mandir, Aurangabad
Tel: 82752 84178

Ashiana Institute for Autism
Nityanand Marg, Municipal
School Ground Floor (Opposite
Garware Plastics) Sahar Road,
Koldongri, Andheri East
Mumbai – 400 069
Tel: 022 – 2684 5062, 2612 5742
Email: ashiana_institute@hotmail.com

La Casa (The School
For Autism and Special
Needs) Ganpati complex
G-2, G-3, Sector- 20, Tong
Apartment, Belapur Village,
Near Ram Mandir Navi Mumbai
Tel: 022 – 6521 0690,
90046 04330
Email: sheena@lacasaschool.com
Web: www.lacasaschool.com

Smt. Radhabai Jamnadas
Thakkar Autistic Centre
Shree Manav Seva Sangh
255-257, Sion Road, Sion (West)
Mumbai–400022
Tel: 022 – 2407 1553,
2407 7350, 2401 5561,
2407 7327
Email: info@shreemanavsevasangh.org
Web: http://www.shreemanavsevasangh.org

Samarpan Centre for Autism
Spectrum

A – 4 Silver Arch Haridas Nagar
Borivali (W) Mumbai 400 057
Tel: 98929 77416, 93232 02768
Email: samarpan@sopan.org
Web: www.sopan.org

SAIRAM Autism Centre
Jai Vakeel Special School
Opposite Milan Industrial Estate
Abhyudaya Nagar
Sewri Hills, Sewri
Mumbai 400 033
Tel: 022–2470 1231, 2470 2285

ASPIRE Educational Services
205AA LBS Marg
Ghatkopar (W) Mumbai
Tel: 99674 85161
Email: aspiedu@gmail.com

Child Development Center
(CDC) at the Hinduja Hospital
Room No. 2310,
2nd floor, OPD building
P.D. Hinduja Hospital, Mahim,
Mumbai–400016
Tel: 022–2445 1515
ext- 8258/ 8259, 2447258/59
Email: vrajeshudani@yahoo.co.in

Umang Charitable Trust
(Special School for Autistics and
Slow Learners)
93/924 Siddhivinayak CHS Ltd.
Off New Link Road, Mahavir
Nagar, Kandivali (W)
Mumbai – 400067
Tel: 022 – 2860 0624
Email: info@umang-trust.org
Web: http://www.umang-trust.
org

Dakshinya Special Education
Centre & School for Autism
A 32/250, Old Siddharth Nagar
Road no. 10, Behind Aadarsha
Vidyalaya Goregaon (W)
Mumbai – 400062
Tel: 98190 23790

Support for Autistic Individuals
(SAI)
201, 2nd Floor Bhagya Ratan
Niwas Above Prabhu Jewellers
3rd Road Khar (W)
Mumbai 400 054
Tel: 022–2605 0992, 2605 0991
Email: saiconnections01@
gmail.com
Web: www.saiconnections.com

Khushi Pediatric Therapy Center,
Bungalow No 6, Manju
Building, Plot No 286-A, Sher-e-
Punjab, Andheri (East),
Mumbai- 400093
Tel: 98195 61468
Email: info@khushi.net.in
Web: http://www.khushi.net.in

Podar Khushi Kids Saraswati
Road Santacruz (W)
Mumbai- 400054
Tel: 022-26465393,
022-26488499
Email: talktous@podar.net
Web: http://podarkhushikids.
com

Priyanj Special School
239/1905 Motilal Nagar No.1,
Achyut Behre Marg, Near
Ganesh Mandir, Road No. 4,

Goregaon (west),
Mumbai – 400104.
Tel: 022 – 2875 3880,
9821098325
Email: info@
priyanjspecialschool.com
Web: priyanjspecialschool.com

Autism Centre
c/o Prasanna Hospital
Deccan Gymkhana,
Pune 411004
Tel: 91–020–25652246
Email: info@prasannaautism.org
Web: http://www.
prasannaautism.org

Sanmvedana School for Children
with Autism
Opposite Landar Park,
Near Hanuman Mandir
Ramdaspeth
Nagpur 400 015
Tel: 3290434, 9822571619,
2284621, 9765290903

Mizoram
Spastics Society of Mizoram
B/68 R Laldanga Building
Chhinga Veng Aizawl 796001

Orissa
Autism Action Group Trust
Flat No.411 Krishna Arcade
Dolamundai
Orissa 751007
Tel: 94373 15517
E-mail: aag.odisha@rediffmail.
com

Centre for Autism Therapy,
Counselling and Help (CATCH)
26, Madhusudan Nagar
Unit 4, Bhubaneswar
Orissa – 751001
Tel: 99370 04040
Email: jenareeta@hotmail.com
Web: http://www.catchindia.org

ARMAAN
N-2/36, IRC Village
Bhubaneshwar
Orissa–751015
Tel: 0674 – 2552030,
95569 34191
Email: armaan@blossomsschool.
in

Punjab
Blue Rose School for Children
with Autism
5, Hargobind Nagar, Sirhind
Road (Opp. Govt. Press)
Patiala – 147004
Tel: 0175–2360958,
93567 67367, 94176 86400
Email: autismindiatoday@gmail.
com, autismindiatoday@yahoo.
com

Darpan
80, Gurdev Nagar Ludhiana
Tel: 94171 60463, 97799 13463
Web: www.darpanautism.org

Sawera
Dr BR Ambedkar Centre
Guru Ravidas Mandir Complex
Opp New Railway Station
Sector 2, Naya Nangal, Ropar

Tel: 01887– 221574,
94170 43267, 94170 43267
Email: sawera_chd@hotmail.com

SOCH- The Autism Society of
Punjab
13, Gujral Nagar Jalandhar City
Tel: 98143 60213,
94634 65208, 98782 11224
E-mail: soch.jal@gmail.com

Sikkim

Spastics society of Sikkim
Special Education and
Rehabilitation Centre Jeewan
Thing Marg Development Area
Gangtok 737101
Tel: 03592 231984
Email: dr-bpdhakal@gmail.com
Web: sikkim.nic.in

Tamil Nadu

We Can Trust
No. 5 Blue Beach Road,
Neelangarai, Chennai 600 041
Tel: 044 – 65461010,
42862221
Email: info@wecanindia.org
Web: www.wecanindia.org

Parents Movement for Autistic
and Intellectually Disabled
(PMAID)
No. 687, HIG II, 3rd Street
Mogappair Lake,
Chennai 600 037
Tel: 044 – 43016712,
98840 02550, 93818 40001
Email: pmaidtrust@gmail.com,
info@maansamithra.org

Web: maansamithra.org

AIKYA New7, Bhagirathi Street
R.A Puram, Chennai 600028
Tel: 044 – 2493 8443,
2461 2668, 94449 60643
Email: info@aikya.org
Web: www.aikya.org

Swabhimaan – Holistic Solutions
for Autism
Plot No: 218 & 201,
Palkalai Nagar, Palavakkam,
Chennai–600041
Tel: 044 – 24510106,
98411 27599
Email: ism_chhc@hotmail.com
Web:
http://www.autismchennai.in

Sankalp Learning Centre
No.4, Sathalwar Street(End
of Paneer Nagar Main Road)
Mogappair West
Chennai 600037 Tamil Nadu
Tel: 044 – 26520062
Email: sindhu.kumar@
sankalpnet.org
Web: sankalpnet.org

Vidial Groups
Vidial Rehabilitation Center
2/46, 2nd Main Road,
Kanakasabai Nagar
Chidambaram
Cuddalore District
Tamil Nadu – 608 001
Tel: 4144 – 224970, 99420
32893, 94884 76165
Email: selva@vidialgroups.org,
vidiyalselva@gmail.com

Website: www.vidialgroups.org

Rajasthan

Approach Autism Society
41, Nemi Sagar Vaishali Nagar
Jaipur - 302021
Tel: 0141-6599102,
92143 09551, 99900 22330
Email: approach.autism@gmail.com
Web: www.approach-autism.in

Sambhav Special School for
Autism
28 Kasturba Nagar, Nirman
Nagar
Ajmer Road Malviya Nagar
Jaipur - 302017
Tel: 0141–3139330, 93093
74871, 96802 49165
Email: sambhavjpr@gmail.com

Asha Ka Jharna Harlalka Kothi
Nawalgarh 333042
Tel: 01594–222930, 223094
Email: sudeepgo@rediffmail.com, info@ashakajharna.org
Web: ashakajharna.org

Uttar Pradesh

Well Being Special School
218, Gyan Khand-1st
Indirapuram, Ghaziabad
UP 201010
Tel: 0120–2691296,
6583395, 98119 58619
Email: drritavats26@yahoo.co.in
Web: www.wellbeingspecial.in

Parents Network for Autism
C-213, Patel Park Nirala Nagar

Lucknow- 226020
Tel: 0522 – 2786508

Muskan Special Education
Centre for Autism
M.S. 39, Sec-D (Near Puraniya
Chauraha), Aliganj, Lucknow
Tel: 0522 – 2334811,
97949 04682

Uttarakhand

Hopes Centre for Autism and
Developmental Disabilitites
99/2 Chakrata Road Adjacent
to NIIT Dehradun 248001
Tel: 97 19 193401

U.S.R Indu Samiti
Village- Basal P.O Peerumadara
Ramnagar
District Nainital 244715
Tel: 99173 42822
Email: usrindusociety@gmail.com
Web: www.usrindusociety.org

West Bengal

Autism Society West Bengal
22 Anjuman Ara Begum Row
Kolkata 700 033
Tel: 033 – 6458 1576,
98301 39173
Email: autismsocietywb@gmail.com
Web: autismsocietywb.org

Parent Circle Time Autism
Identified (PACTAI)
Mrs.Krishna Roy (Principal)
Alokdhara
47C/1Dharmatala Road

Kolkata 700 042
Tel: 033 – 64508205, 99038 45071
E-mail: query@alokdhara-inclusion.org
Web: alokdhara-inclusion.org

Creating Connections
10/4 Block B
6 Sunny Park
Kolkata – 700019

Tel: 98309 41233, 98102 25923
Email: shaneelm@gmail.com

Pradip (Centre for Autism Management)
203B Lake Town, Block B
Kolkata – 700089
Tel: 033 – 2534 1832, 2534 0891, 93310 47831
Web: pradipautism.org

Disclaimer

The addresses, phone numbers, email ids of the above organizations might have changed. The author and the publisher are not responsible for the changes.

Autism Internet Groups Related to India

1. India Developmental Disabilities – This is a friendly supportive group which discusses daily challenges of raising a child with developmental disabilities. The group's mission is to support and help each other.

Support group.

https://groups.yahoo.com/neo/groups/India_DevelopmentalDisabilities/info

2. Autism India Network – This is a platform to discuss about early intervention and the different approaches in training the children affected with Autistic Spectrum Disorder.

https://in.groups.yahoo.com/neo/groups/AutismIndia/info

Request to the readers

Please fill in the feedback form and help us to guide the autism community.

Feedback Form of Autism Book

1) Age of the child _____
2) State/Union Territory you live in _____
3) Are you a parent/relative/teacher/therapist etc.? _____
4) What did you like about the book? _____
   _____
5) What would you like to include in the next edition of this book? _____
6) Any other suggestion/comment _____
   _____
   _____

Please send the feedback form to–

V & S Publishers

F – 2/16 Ansari Road Daryaganj New Delhi - 110002

You may even email the feedback at
info@vspublishers.com.

Please write "Autism feedback" in the subject line.

Look at autism through your heart

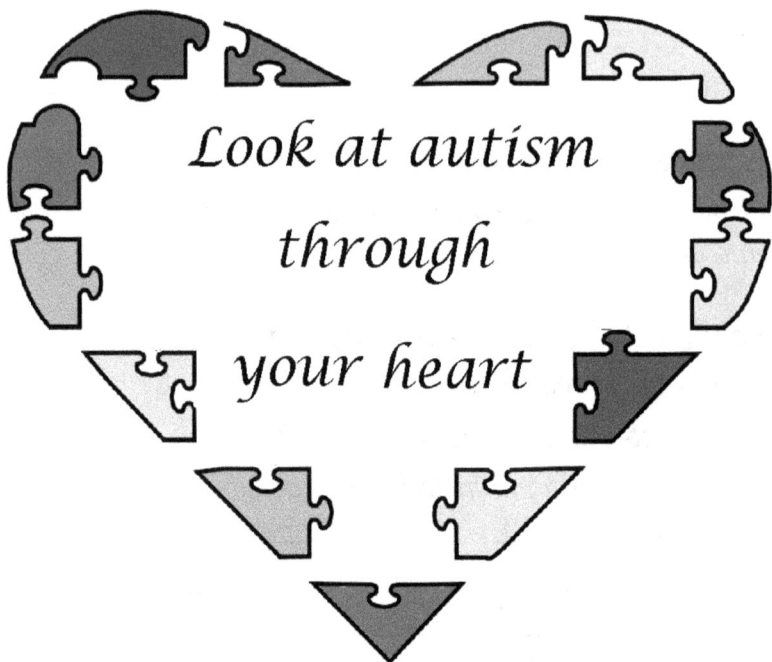

A child is just a floating butterfly
  Etching out patterns in the air,
Each hovering to their best
Comparing one to other is not fair.
In their uniqueness lies their beauty,
To bring out their potential is our duty.

By
Parthasarathi Mitra

www.ingramcontent.com/pod-product-compliance
Lightning Source LLC
Chambersburg PA
CBHW050717280326
41926CB00088B/3110